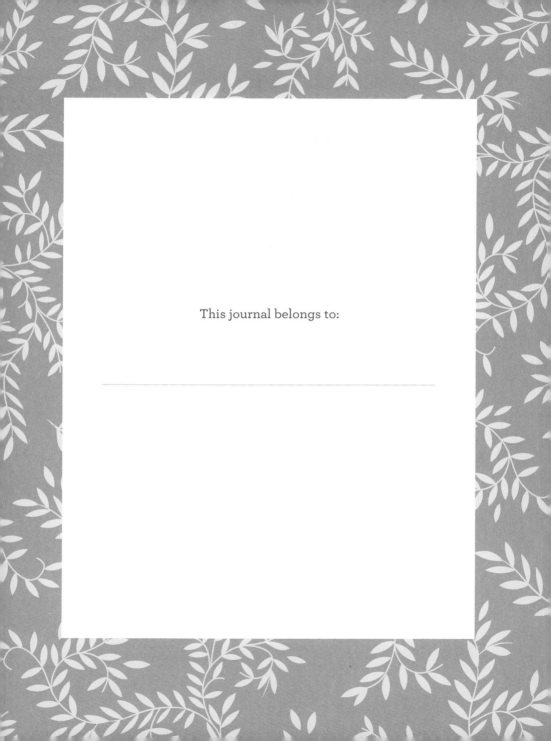

This journal belongs to:

_____

# Journaling
## Through Your
# Pregnancy

# Journaling
## Through Your
# Pregnancy

Devotions and Prayers for Each Week
of Your Baby's Development

Jennifer Polimino and Carolyn Warren

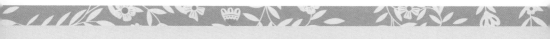

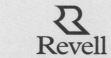

Revell
*a division of Baker Publishing Group*
**Grand Rapids, Michigan**

Published by Revell
a division of Baker Publishing Group
Grand Rapids, Michigan
RevellBooks.com

Printed in China

Library of Congress Cataloging-in-Publication Control Number: 2024021525

ISBN 9780800746438 (cloth)
ISBN 9781493447237 (ebook)

Unless otherwise indicated, Scripture quotations are from the Holman Christian Standard Bible®. Copyright © 1999, 2000, 2002, 2003, 2009 by Holman Bible Publishers. Used by permission. Holman Christian Standard Bible®, Holman CSB®, and HCSB® are federally registered trademarks of Holman Bible Publishers.

Scripture quotations labeled ESV are from The Holy Bible, English Standard Version® (ESV®). Copyright © 2001 by Crossway, a publishing ministry of Good News Publishers. Used by permission. All rights reserved. ESV Text Edition: 2016

Scripture quotations labeled GW are from GOD'S WORD®. Copyright © 1995, 2003, 2013, 2014, 2019, 2020 by God's Word to the Nations Mission Society. Used by permission.

Scripture quotations labeled KJV are from the King James Version of the Bible.

Scripture quotations labeled NIV are from the Holy Bible, New International Version®, NIV®. Copyright © 1973, 1978, 1984, 2011 by Biblica, Inc.® Used by permission of Zondervan. All rights reserved worldwide. www.zondervan.com. The "NIV" and "New International Version" are trademarks registered in the United States Patent and Trademark Office by Biblica, Inc.®

Scripture quotations labeled NKJV are from the New King James Version®. Copyright © 1982 by Thomas Nelson. Used by permission. All rights reserved.

Scripture quotations labeled NLT are from the Holy Bible, New Living Translation. Copyright © 1996, 2004, 2015 by Tyndale House Foundation. Used by permission of Tyndale House Publishers, Carol Stream, Illinois 60188. All rights reserved.

Portions of this text have been taken from *Praying Through Your Pregnancy* by Jennifer Polimino and Carolyn Warren, published by Revell, 2024.

This publication is intended to provide helpful and informative material on the subjects addressed. Readers should consult their personal health professionals before adopting any of the suggestions in this book or drawing inferences from it. The author and publisher expressly disclaim responsibility for any adverse effects arising from the use or application of the information contained in this book.

Cover design: Laura Klynstra
Interior book design by Nadine Rewa

24  25  26  27  28  29  30      7  6  5  4  3  2  1

# Contents

## Third Trimester: Weeks 28 to Birth

# Introduction

Dear Sweet Friend,

You are embarking upon the amazing journey into motherhood. Before you know it, your baby will arrive, and you will be holding your little child in your arms and looking deeply into his or her eyes. Some of you have waited a very long time to get pregnant, and others of you may already have children. Whether this is your first baby or your fourth, I pray that *Journaling Through Your Pregnancy* will be a blessing to you and someday to your child, as you can gift this journal to your child as a keepsake.

My hope is that this book will guide and encourage you to dig deep within your heart and answer the questions each day with sincerity. Please take your time as you journal, for this book will become a treasure to your child someday to look back on and read exactly what you were going through while you were pregnant with him or her.

I also pray that you allow the Holy Spirit to be your Helper while you are pregnant. He is your Counselor, your Advocate, and your compassionate Friend. He is your Healer and your Redeemer. He wants to fill you with peace and joy and speak to you in His still small voice.

So I encourage you to be filled with the Holy Spirit throughout the next 41 weeks and beyond. Did you know that to be filled with the Holy Spirit is a command? Our obedience rests strictly on our choice to obey what the Father tells us to do. When we choose to obey Him, we are the ones who benefit.

If you are at all doubting if Jesus' Spirit lives inside you, I encourage you to make sure right now. Let's take a moment and humbly ask the Lord to come inside you today.

All you need to do first is to acknowledge that you have sinned before the Lord (Rom. 3:23). Next, confess any sins that come to mind and lay them before the feet of Jesus, and He will forgive you (1 John 1:9). Repent of your sin and stop doing it. Acts 3:19 says that if we repent and turn to God, our sins will be wiped out. Then invite Jesus' Spirit to come inside you and live in you (Rev. 3:20). Now it's time to give control of your life to Him (Acts 2:36). Last, you are encouraged to share the good news with another person and let them know that you are publicly declaring that Jesus lives inside you (Rom. 10:9–10).

Now that you have prayed this, the Holy Spirit dwells within you, and He will be walking with you during your entire pregnancy journey. Hallelujah! If this was the first time that you asked Jesus into your heart, I am celebrating and rejoicing with you. Praise the Lord!

If you prayed this prayer today, please send me a note (Jen@PrayFor YourBaby.com) so I can pray for you and speak a blessing over you and your baby.

Okay, now you're ready to get started on your pregnancy journal. Let's dive into week 1.

# First Trimester

# Weeks 1–12

This is the word of the Lᴏʀᴅ
your Maker who formed you from the womb;
He will help you.

Isaiah 44:2

> Trust in the LORD with all your heart,
> and do not rely on your own understanding;
> think about Him in all your ways,
> and He will guide you on the right paths.
>
> Proverbs 3:5–6

Your baby is special to God, even before he or she is conceived. This makes perfect sense, because God isn't bound by time like we are, and He can see straight into the future. He knows all about your baby beforehand—what he or she will look like, what he'll like and dislike, what her special talents will be. More importantly, God has a plan for your baby's life, and you can trust Him with all your heart.

A boy named Jeremiah was called by God to be a leader even before his father and mother conceived him. You might wonder, is that a fantasy, or does God really see babies before they are conceived? Look at what God said in Jeremiah 1:5: "I chose you before I formed you in the womb; I set you apart before you were born. I appointed you a prophet to the nations."

History tells us that when Jeremiah grew up, he foretold of God's judgment and the overthrow of Jerusalem, the 70 years of captivity and the promise of restoration of the Jews—fulfilling God's promise that Jeremiah would be a prophet to the nations.

## Your Baby's Name Is on God's Calendar

Could your baby have a plan designed by God for his or her life, even before he or she is born? Yes, absolutely. The possibilities are intriguing. Your child may be called to be an evangelist, teacher, music leader, inventor, financier, or writer. God sees into the future, and He knows what plans He has for your child. Acts 17:24–27 tells us that God made the world and everything in it, that He Himself gives everyone life and breath and has determined our appointed times. Does that strike you like it strikes me? God gives babies life and breath in His appointed time—it's like your baby's birth date is written on God's calendar and He's got the date circled in pink or blue! Another Scripture that confirms this concept is Ephesians 1:4: "For He chose us in Him, before the foundation of the world." Can you imagine that? You are waiting anxiously for a positive pregnancy test, and God's Word says He has already chosen your child way back before the foundation of the world!

Lord, this week, I am feeling and thinking about:

_____

_____

_____

_____

_____

_____

What are You saying to me?

_____

_____

_____

_____

_____

_____

What I most look forward to with this baby:

_____

_____

_____

_____

_____

_____

Jesus, right now I'm struggling with:

_____

_____

_____

_____

_____

_____

This week, I am praying for this child to:

_____

_____

_____

_____

_____

_____

This week, I release to God my cares and concerns about:

_____

_____

_____

_____

_____

_____

_____

## A Mother's Prayer for Week 1

Dear Lord,

I believe You have a divine plan for each of our lives. You know the future, and You know the child I am going to have, even now. Jeremiah 1:5 says, "I chose you before I formed you in the womb." I take this as an encouragement that You see into the future and You know all about this new life.

You know all things, and You are still doing miracles today. I agree with Your Word, and I command stress, anxiety, and worry to go, in the name of Jesus. Instead, I will choose to meditate on Your promises.

I receive Your peace. Philippians 4:7 says, "The peace of God, which surpasses every thought, will guard your hearts and minds in Christ Jesus." I thank You for peace.

Lord, help me be the best mother I can be. Give me the wisdom to raise this child according to Your ways, so that he or she grows to love You and serve You all his or her life. I thank You for the good plans for me and my family. My future and my hope are in You and You alone.

In Jesus' name I pray. Amen.

# Week 2

Don't you know that your body is a sanctuary of the Holy Spirit who is in you, whom you have from God? You are not your own, for you were bought at a price. Therefore glorify God in your body.

1 Corinthians 6:19–20

When you're pregnant or soon-to-be pregnant, it's important to treat your body with care and respect, because you are bringing a new life into the world, and this little person is totally dependent on you for his or her health. This is an awesome responsibility. I encourage you to take it seriously and to ask God for His help.

Even if you have a history of bad habits, such as eating unhealthy foods and ignoring exercise, you can turn that around now by making a commitment and claiming God's promise in Philippians 4:13: "I am able to do all things through Him who strengthens me." So no matter where you are right now in your physical and spiritual health, this is the perfect time for you to soar ahead to new heights—using good principles of health, prayer, and reliance on God's strength. Here are five important tips to help you during your pregnancy too.

1. **Support your pregnancy with proper nutrition.** Expectant moms need about 340 more calories a day for a single birth and 600 calories for twins.[1] Don't fall into the trap of thinking, *I'm going to gain weight anyway, so this is my chance to eat whatever I feel like eating.* Choose healthy options—everything you put into your body goes to your baby too. You'll need 75–100 grams of protein a day, critical for growth and your baby's brain cells. Fruits and vegetables high in vitamin C help your baby's bone and tooth development and manufacture collagen, which holds tissue together and helps in delivery. Carbohydrates provide necessary fuel for your body and your baby's body and have been known to help with morning sickness.

2. **Take folate (folic acid) and prenatal vitamins now.** Your baby needs folate from the very beginning, and multivitamins ensure that you and your baby get all the key nutrients you need.

3. **Form a water habit.** Aim for at least eight glasses of water a day. Guard against dehydration.

4. **Exercise as you are able.** It's magnificent for building strength and flexibility, which you will need during labor and when your little one arrives. It is also helpful for relieving stress and coping with wild mood swings caused by pregnancy hormones. Make sure you follow your physician's recommendation for exercise. Every woman and pregnancy is unique, so exercise only according to what is healthy and safe for you.

5. **Rest, rest, rest.** Sleep, sleep, sleep. Don't feel bad about craving sleep. It's perfectly normal.

Now is a good time to find new joy in taking good care of your body, knowing that you are respecting the perfect vessel God gave to you to carry your baby.

Lord, this week, I am feeling and thinking about:

_____

_____

_____

_____

_____

_____

What are You saying to me?

_____

_____

_____

_____

_____

_____

I commit to taking care of my body as God's vessel by:

I want my child to learn about living a healthy lifestyle from me. Here's what I pray for my child's life:

_____

_____

_____

_____

_____

This week, I release to God my cares and concerns about:

_____

_____

_____

_____

_____

## A Mother's Prayer for Week 2

Dear Lord,

Help me to respect the body that You gave me. I make a commitment today to treat it right by following principles of good nutrition and by exercising. Your Word says the body is the sanctuary of the Holy Spirit; help me treat my body with the care it deserves. Be my strength and motivation, God, for "I am able to do all things through Him who strengthens me" (Phil. 4:13).

I will look to You for a healthy self-image, Lord. I will not give in to binge eating, overeating, or starvation diets. I will look to you for a healthy lifestyle, which includes rest and sleep. John 8:32 says, "You will know the truth, and the truth will set you free." I claim this promise for myself, and that I will be free of all ungodly, unhealthy eating habits.

I pray for good health for myself and for my baby, and to reflect a Christian witness in all I do.

In Jesus' name. Amen.

# Week 3

Acknowledge that Yahweh is God.
He made us, and we are His.

Psalm 100:3

Something of major importance happened in that very first second when you became pregnant. God chose the sex of your baby. Can you imagine what that means? At that very moment, even before there is a head and body or a recognizable shape, there is a male or female in the making.

One cell of life, just one second old . . . and yet so much is already determined.

Within hours of conception, that single cell formed by your X and the daddy's Y or X has divided again and again. Just a few days later, this microscopic bundle of cells, which is about one-fifth the size of the dot over the letter *i*, is cruising through your fallopian tube to the warm, nourishing space that will be his or her internal nursery—your uterus. Once there, it takes about six days for your newly conceived baby to settle in and start getting nourishment from you through your bloodstream. Everything you eat—from that nutritious green salad to those fat-soaked, salt-drenched fries—is going into the tiny baby that is doing his or her best to grow and be healthy.

Something else is happening too. Your baby takes in the nutrition and releases the human chorionic gonadotropin (HCG) hormone into your bloodstream. This can cause all kinds of surprises—you're suddenly zapped of energy and want to take naps, or you can no longer stand certain smells, or your stomach turns inside out, or you feel hyperemotional and get into an argument with someone you love over the tiniest, most unimportant thing.

And then it dawns on you. *Could it be? Could I be pregnant?*

If you haven't already begun, now is the time to start praying for your pregnancy and your baby. Prayer is ordained by God, and we are instructed in the Holy Bible to pray. Even Jesus, God's only Son, the Anointed One, prayed to His Heavenly Father, and He intercedes for us. The Bible tells us that Jesus is interceding for us in Heaven before the Father: "Therefore he is able, once and forever, to save those who come to God through him. He lives forever to intercede with God on their behalf" (Heb. 7:25 NLT).

The book of Ephesians tells us to pray at all times in the Spirit (Eph. 6:18). But how can we possibly pray all the time when we live a busy life and are getting ready for a new baby? Well, God says that He hears our prayers, but He can also read our thoughts. So we can be washing dishes, preparing meals, or changing a diaper, and be talking to God in our minds about the child growing inside of us.

I believe that God wants mothers today, more than ever, to begin praying for their sons and daughters right from the very start—even before they are born. God has given you as the parent the authority to claim the biblical promises on your baby's behalf. You have the power to give him or her the advantage of prayer starting right now.

Lord, this week, I am feeling and thinking about:

_____

_____

_____

_____

_____

_____

What are You saying to me?

_____

_____

_____

_____

_____

_____

_____

Jesus, this week, I pray for joy for the unique baby that God is creating within me. This is my prayer:

_____

_____

_____

_____

_____

_____

_____

_____

_____

_____

I am guessing that my child is a (circle one):

boy          girl

This week, I release to God my cares and concerns about:

## A Mother's Prayer for Week 3

Dear Heavenly Father,

Thank You for the child You are giving me. Thank You for the awesome miracle of new life. You are the only one who knows if I am having a boy or a girl. I ask You to bless my baby with good health and with love.

Help me to feel well physically, and take away any morning sickness or other hardships that may make it hard for me to concentrate on You and this amazing gift You are giving me.

I pray against miscarriage, Jesus. I know how common it is, but I am trusting You for a healthy baby.

In Jesus' name. Amen.

# Week 4

Who has put wisdom in the mind?
Or who has given understanding to the heart?
                                        Job 38:36 NKJV

Your baby is just 14 days old, and yet something of monumental importance is happening. A sheet of cells is rapidly growing into what will become your baby's brain, spinal cord, and backbone. Why these three? The answer is fascinating.

The brain is going to control everything your child does—from involuntary breathing, to talking, to balancing on a bicycle and learning to read. Although the brain gives instructions to the body, it can't do its job alone; it needs a long bundle of nerves to relay messages to (and from) the various parts of the body. These tireless "message senders" are located inside the spinal column, which is protected by the vertebrae. It's a complex and beautiful design engineered by our Creator God.

Your baby's placenta and umbilical cord have already been forming as well. Don't be surprised if you feel like sleeping more than usual. You might find yourself out of your normal routine, and that's okay, because once your new baby comes, your routine is going to be interrupted a lot! However, some women don't feel sick or tired or any different at all during their first weeks of pregnancy, and if that's the case for you, don't worry— consider yourself blessed. Every pregnancy is unique, just as God made each of us unique.

The one thing we can all do as moms and moms-to-be is to pray for our babies now. I suggest you have a regular time of day for praying, because when prayer becomes part of your routine, you don't forget. Some people like to say a short prayer as soon as they wake up, even before they get out of bed. You might look at the clock and say, "Thank You, Lord, for this day. I believe You're going to help me make it a wonderful day. Lead me and guide me and use me today for Your kingdom and Your glory, and please bless my baby. In Jesus' name. Amen." This way, you get up knowing that the Holy Spirit is right with you. There's no "getting up on the wrong side of the bed" when you start your day with Jesus!

Along with the fact that at some point in the pregnancy your baby can hear your voice, I believe that your baby also bonds with you even before he or she is born by becoming accustomed to your voice. Although your baby probably can't hear you clearly yet, it's good to get in the habit of audible prayer. I also like to pray out loud because hearing the prayers that incorporate the power of God's Word bolsters my faith. So even though God can hear your thoughts, I recommend praying aloud sometimes too. When you speak aloud God's truth through prayer, you release the power of God to work in your life. And as you hear yourself speak, your faith is strengthened as well. When you grasp the realization that you can tap into our divine Resource through prayer, you understand the power you have at your disposal. God wants you to use this power to bring His will to pass in your life.

Lord, this week, I am feeling and thinking about:

_____

_____

_____

_____

_____

_____

What are You saying to me?

_____

_____

_____

_____

_____

_____

I want to hear Your voice, Lord. And I want my baby to learn from me how to listen to Your voice. I am listening. What are You saying to me today?

This week, I release to God my cares and concerns about:

_____

_____

_____

_____

_____

_____

_____

_____

_____

_____

_____

_____

_____

_____

_____

## A Mother's Prayer for Week 4

Dear Lord,

Thank You for this baby growing inside me. I can't quite understand what is going on with my baby at this moment, so I give him or her to You and ask for Your blessing. Lord, please help my baby's brain develop perfectly, and give my baby wisdom beyond his or her years.

God, You are the Creator of all life. I pray now that this baby will grow according to Your plan for my pregnancy. I pray that the cells will multiply and grow and that the brain and spinal cord will develop properly. Give my baby a strong spinal cord and a strong, intelligent mind.

Please bless my baby's growth and make my baby healthy and strong.

I pray that my son or daughter will grow up to be a person of prayer—that he or she will have faith and tap into Your power through prayer.

In Jesus' name. Amen.

# Week 5

I encourage you to call your family and friends and ask them to commit to joining you in praying for your baby throughout your pregnancy.

By five weeks, your baby's heart has started beating. Your doctor probably won't hear it with a stethoscope yet, but ultrasound machines have detected movement of a baby's heart at this point in the pregnancy. Just think, God hears your baby's heart beating! Remember, God said He knows us before we're born, and He is very much aware of the baby growing rapidly inside you.

By next week, your baby's heart will beat about 150 times a minute and remain at that rate until birth. After your baby is born, the heart pumps blood to every cell in the body in less than 60 seconds, every second for a lifetime. Just how many heartbeats does that add up to? One estimate, based on averages, is 2.8 billion heartbeats.[1] Now that's what I call an example of God's creative power!

Perhaps you are worried that when it's time to hear your baby's heartbeat, it won't be there. Be encouraged by the story of my friend Darla Sanborn. At her six-week checkup and ultrasound, the physician said, "I'm sorry, Mrs. Sanborn, but you've lost the baby. You will miscarry soon." Darla didn't want to accept that verdict. She felt certain that she was pregnant with a live baby, so she requested a second ultrasound. The verdict remained the same after the second one. Darla was sent home to wait for her body to miscarry her baby.

Instead, Darla went home and prayed and expected her baby to live. She asked her church to join in prayer. Darla's mother and her mother's church also joined in prayer, believing God to turn this verdict around. Darla asked friends to pray, and those friends passed on the prayer request to their churches. She had entire communities of Christians standing in faith for her, proclaiming God's promises in Scripture—praying for her unborn baby.

There is power in receiving the prayer support of others. Jesus said, "Again, I assure you: If two of you on earth agree about any matter that you pray for, it will be done for you by My Father in heaven. For where two or three are gathered together in My name, I am there among them" (Matt. 18:19–20). Darla had many more than two or three praying—so would this make a difference? Darla and her mother had faith that it would.

After two weeks had passed and she still hadn't miscarried, she went to see the ob-gyn in her mother's town. Another ultrasound was performed, and there it was right on the monitor—the baby's heart, beating just as it should. Her baby was alive!

This week, while you're praying for your baby's physical heart, pray also that he or she will grow up with a heart of love for God and others. Jesus said, "I have spoken these things to you so that My joy may be in you and your joy may be complete. This is My command: Love one another as I have loved you" (John 15:11–12).

Loving others with a Christlike love is one way to bring joy into our lives.

Lord, this week, I am feeling and thinking about:

_____

_____

_____

_____

_____

_____

What are You saying to me?

_____

_____

_____

_____

_____

_____

_____

When I think about God using me to create a new life, I:

_____

_____

_____

_____

_____

_____

_____

_____

_____

_____

_____

_____

_____

_____

_____

This week, I release to God my cares and concerns about:

## A Mother's Prayer for Week 5

Dear Father God,

Thank You for this wonderful miracle of life You have given me. May joy and gladness fill my heart and spill over to everyone who hears the good news of my pregnancy. A new baby is a blessing for the whole family, so I pray that our parents will be blessed by the news of this grandbaby. I pray that the uncles, aunties, and cousins will be blessed and filled with joy. And for all our friends and loved ones, let them share in our joy and gratitude. I pray that this time of rejoicing and gladness would also be a time of praising You for Your blessing of the miracle of life. Your Word says that every good and perfect gift comes from above, so I give You my thanks for this wonderful gift.

I thank You for my baby's heartbeat, and even though I can't hear it yet, I know You can. Bless my baby's heart and cause it to grow strong, just as it should be. Protect it from any defects or problems. Your Word says that in the beginning, Your creative powers were at work. I acknowledge Your power and ask You to extend it to my baby also. Create a healthy baby, week by week, as he or she grows.

And Lord, give my child a heart to love and serve You. Give my child a tender heart that's open to hearing Your voice, and help him or her to be kind and compassionate toward others. Please help me to be a good role model of these attitudes. Help me lead my child in prayer and in opening up our hearts to You to receive Your love.

In Jesus' name I pray. Amen.

# Week 6

Call to Me and I will answer you and tell you great and incomprehensible things you do not know.

Jeremiah 33:3

By the end of this week, you will officially have been pregnant for one month—and your baby has grown to triple the size. He or she is now about a quarter inch long, or about the size of a lentil. Still tiny, but your baby's facial features are already beginning to take shape, and much more.

Your baby is taking after you or dad, or a little of both, all according to the directions spelled out in the unique combination of genes you've both provided. Here's what's going on:

- The beginning of eyes and ears are developing with the openings in just the right places.
- A tiny space for the mouth is appearing.
- Your baby's stomach and lungs are beginning to form.
- Small buds that will grow into arms and legs are taking shape.

Talk about a growth spurt! Don't feel bad if you're still craving sleep.

This week, pray for the magnificent growth that is taking place in your baby and, specifically, for the development of self-respect that will be manifested in the facial expression your child portrays to the world—a first impression he or she will project throughout life. When children are young, you can see how they're feeling just by looking at their faces. A toddler doesn't hide a pout or a feeling of sheer delight. It's only as we get older that we learn to mask our feelings.

When we meet someone, one of the first things we usually do is judge that person by his or her face. Our idea of that individual's personality and sense of self often happens in a millisecond impression of his or her facial expression. Think of someone whose face presents a strong sense of self-respect, of someone who has a face that portrays self-confidence regardless of "beauty" or lack of it. Perhaps an image that comes to mind is an older relative, such as a grandmother. She may be 80 years old, with a vast web of lines and creases on her face, and yet she portrays self-respect that manifests to the world an attractive self-confidence.

Pray for everything that's happening with your baby's development this week, especially for the reflection of inner strength—honor and self-respect—that will be manifested on your baby's face for all the world to see. We know God answers prayer.

Lord, this week, I am feeling and thinking about:

_____

_____

_____

_____

_____

_____

What are You saying to me?

_____

_____

_____

_____

_____

_____

_____

These are the character qualities I desire for my child:

I model (or will model) honor and self-respect by:

This week, I release to God my cares and concerns about:

_____

_____

_____

_____

_____

_____

_____

_____

_____

_____

_____

_____

_____

_____

_____

## A Mother's Prayer for Week 6

Dear Lord,

I am so amazed at the miracle of life that's growing inside me. So much is happening for my baby this week. I ask that You watch over him or her and cause the development to go just the way it should. Lord, I pray for my baby's face—the eyes, ears, nose, and mouth. Let the face grow perfectly, just the way it's supposed to. Form those features in a way that will reveal inner strength and outer love. And I pray for the internal parts—the stomach and lungs, the heart and brain. Let them develop into strong, healthy parts for my baby. And last, I pray for the arms and legs to grow just right. Bless my baby in every way: physically, mentally, and spiritually. Give my baby a pure, kind heart and a good soul, open to Your Holy Spirit and to loving You.

I pray that my child will have a healthy sense of self-respect and honor. Help me to teach my child these values and be a good role model of respect and honor toward others. Lord, as a family, we want to portray a Christlike spirit and earn the respect of our community and be a good representative for You.

Once again, I thank You for this wonderful miracle.

In Jesus' name I pray. Amen.

# Week 7

Don't be surprised if you want a nap more than you want to do anything else. This week, your baby is about the size of a blueberry and 10,000 times larger than at conception—and your body is making that happen.

Not only is your baby growing at hyperspeed, but he or she is also generating new brain cells at the mind-boggling rate of 100 cells per minute. By the time your baby is born, he or she will have about 100 billion neurons, which are the nerve cells that speed messages to and from the brain at the rate of up to 200 miles per hour. And something else has been happening. Your baby has developed and gone through three sets of kidneys already, and now he or she has the final set of kidneys—the ones that will remain with him or her for life. We don't often think about our kidneys, but we have to appreciate the service they provide.

The kidneys are sophisticated reprocessing machines designed by God for the important task of filtering out the garbage, and they are at work, even now, while your baby is still developing. In addition, kidneys release three hormones that do the following:

- stimulate bone marrow to make red blood cells
- regulate blood pressure
- help maintain calcium for bones and normal chemical balance in the body

Even though your baby has kidneys, they won't be visible for several more weeks. If you have an ultrasound at week 16 or thereafter, one of the things on the list of items to be examined will be the kidneys.

In order to be healthy, we need a spiritual garbage filter as well. We want our children to filter out the garbage in this world: the things that carry wrong concepts and ideas to their mind and lies of all kinds. We have all sinned and come short of the glory of God, but when we confess our sins, He wipes them away, and it's like having a clean slate (see Rom. 3:23; 1 John 1:9). It's fantastic to know that we can claim victory over every area of temptation, in the name of Jesus.

Pray for your child to be wise as a serpent and harmless as a dove (see Matt. 10:16), to be knowing and yet innocent of evil. There is so much deception in these days that we live in. The Bible is clear that we are not to be deceived, so let's pray for our children to be filled with wisdom and discernment. There's power in praying protection over your unborn baby.

Lord, this week, I am feeling and thinking about:

_____

_____

_____

_____

_____

_____

What are You saying to me?

_____

_____

_____

_____

_____

_____

My ideas for protecting my child from ungodly influences:

_____

_____

_____

_____

_____

_____

_____

_____

_____

_____

_____

_____

_____

_____

_____

This week, I release to God my cares and concerns about:

## A Mother's Prayer for Week 7

Dear God, our wonderful Creator,

I pray for my baby's permanent kidneys that are growing this week. I pray for healthy organs, now and all throughout my child's lifetime, that he or she would never experience kidney failure. Let those kidneys function just as they should, filtering out impurities and releasing hormones the body needs.

I also pray for spiritual purity for my baby. Help me, as the mom, and help my child to filter out all the evil that is in this world. Help me teach my child to love what is good and shun what is evil. Protect my child from pornography and from spiritually damaging media. Open my spiritual eyes so that I will discern what's harmful and keep it out of our home.

Give my child a love for what is righteous and pure and holy. Fill our hearts with so much love for Your Word and for You that we are not drawn into temptation by enticing worldly things. Hebrews 4:12 says that Your Word is alive and powerful and sharper than a two-edged sword; so, Lord, I pray that Your Word will be always in our minds to combat evil. I also ask that You fill me with Your Holy Spirit to empower me, just as You promised in Acts to empower me to live a pure and holy life, so that I can teach my children to live a pure and holy life as well.

In Jesus' name I pray. Amen.

# Week 8

> For when he sees his children,
> the work of My hands within his nation,
> they will honor My name,
> they will honor the Holy One of Jacob
> and stand in awe of the God of Israel.
>
> Isaiah 29:23

When your baby is born, one of the first things the medical staff does is count his or her fingers and toes, and most parents do the same. It's a good feeling when you count to ten and see they're all there. They're so cute! I don't know anybody who doesn't marvel at how exquisite a newborn baby's hands are.

Science tells us the fingertips have one of the highest concentrations of temperature and touch receptors among all areas of the skin, making them extremely sensitive to heat, cold, moisture, texture, pressure, and vibration. Your baby will use these sensory probes to discover the world around him or her. He or she will learn to catch a ball, comb his or her hair, pet a cat, and color a picture without consciously maneuvering the fingers. Perhaps you never thought about it before, but when you decide to pick up a mug and pour yourself some coffee, you don't have to think about what your fingers are doing—the movements are unconscious.

So many special skills and talents that God gives us involve using the hands and fingers—from rebuilding an engine to creating beautiful calligraphy to decorating a cake. Maybe it's playing football, and you'll be teaching your child how to throw a pass. Or sharing a big box of crayons and coloring with your child. Pray that whatever special gifts God blesses your baby with, these gifts will be used for the glory of the Lord.

Pray for your baby's hands, that he or she would use them to help others and always show love. Pray that your child will not cause harm with his or her hands, that they would be strong but gentle. Ask God to bless those hands and use them for His glory, that your child will make beautiful music for worship and praise. Whatever it will be, pray for your baby's hands and ask God for what you desire for your child.

This week, the elbows and wrists are developing, and your baby may even start flexing them. In addition, his or her main internal organs continue to grow stronger. And your baby's feet and toes are beginning to form, which is a good reminder to share your desire with God that your child will walk with Christ all the days of his or her life, no matter where those feet take him or her.

Lord, this week, I am feeling and thinking about:

_____

_____

_____

_____

_____

_____

What are You saying to me?

_____

_____

_____

_____

_____

_____

A blessing for my baby:

This week, I release to God my cares and concerns about:

_____

_____

_____

_____

_____

_____

_____

_____

_____

_____

_____

_____

_____

## A Mother's Prayer for Week 8

Dear Lord,

I pray for my baby's hands and fingers, feet and toes, that they will grow and develop properly. I pray for the elbows and wrists that are developing as well, that they will be good and strong and flex as they should.

Please bless my baby's hands and use them for the good of Your kingdom. Bless my baby's feet and help my child to always walk with You, God.

Lord, I thank You for blessing each one of us with special gifts and talents. I pray that whatever my child does with his or her hands, he or she will do it well and use it for building Your kingdom. Bless the work of my child's hands. Help him or her to be diligent in that work so he or she may be viewed as having godly character. And, Lord, bless my child's feet that they might go where You want them to go, for Your ministry.

I know that every good and perfect gift comes from above, and I acknowledge You as our Creator and God. I praise You for all You have done and for all You will do.

In Jesus' name. Amen.

# Week 9

Test me, Lᴏʀᴅ, and try me;
examine my heart and mind.

Psalm 26:2

When I was born in Oak Park, Illinois, I had just one sibling at the time, an older sister. Originally, my parents planned on having only two children, but that soon changed. When I was almost three years old, my parents had enough of the frigid winters and scorching summers in Chicago, so they loaded me, my sister, and my new baby brother into a motor home to search for a more desirable place to raise their family. From June until early September, we cruised across 43 states. Although we saw many beautiful sites, including the Rocky Mountains and Grand Canyon, my parents didn't find what they were looking for, so they packed us up again the following summer, and we flew to the South Pacific. We traveled all throughout Tahiti, Samoa, Fiji, and Hawaii. We were on 24 flights in three and a half months.

My parents fell in love with Hawaii and liked the fact that it was part of the United States, so they returned to Chicago, sold everything, and flew back to Hawaii. Mom and Dad bought a small house overlooking Kailua-Kona Bay and made it into a loving home. We attended a church there on the Big Island of Hawaii called Calvary Community Church.

In spite of my parents' original idea to have just two children, our family grew to nine, including my mom and dad. It always was an exciting time in the house when we were planning for the next baby to arrive. God bestowed my mom with a special gift—mothering!

We had fun and wild times growing up. There was always something going on: a Bible study at our house, a group outing, or a church potluck. Now I can look back and see what a truly great life my parents gave us. There were hard times too, but I always knew that I was loved by my family and by God. The overall heartbeat of our family was healthy and strong.

My parents taught us that talking to God and trusting Him should be part of our daily lives.

Now jump ahead about 38 years to the day we went to see our second baby's ultrasound. Both my husband and I felt the same way—we didn't care if it was a boy or a girl; we just wanted a healthy baby with a good, strong heart. I thought back to growing up in Hawaii in a large family, and I knew there were certain things about the heart of that family that I wanted to carry over into my own family now. A sense of belonging, the way we knew our parents cared for us, and the pursuit of godly ideals—those were all things I wanted for my children too.

When you hear your baby's heartbeat for the first time, I hope you experience God's presence with you and know that you've been blessed with a wonderful gift. And I hope you take some time to think about the heartbeat of your own family and what that means to you. What makes your family special? What bonds you together? How can you invite Jesus Christ to be a central part of your lives?

If you don't hear your baby's heartbeat this week, don't panic. It's probably because your baby is snuggling in a cozy corner of your uterus or has his or her back facing out, making it difficult to pick up the sound. In a week or so, you'll probably have the joy of hearing the fast-paced *thump-thump* of your baby's heart.

Lord, this week, I am feeling and thinking about:

What are You saying to me?

What it was like when I heard my baby's heartbeat for the first time:

This week, I release to God my cares and concerns about:

_____

_____

_____

_____

_____

_____

_____

_____

_____

_____

_____

_____

_____

_____

## A Mother's Prayer for Week 9

Dear Lord,

Thank You for this special person growing inside of me. I pray that this time of rejoicing and gladness would also be a time of praising You for Your blessing of the miracle of life. Your Word says that every good and perfect gift comes from above, so I give You my thanks for this wonderful gift.

I pray that my baby grows to be a man or woman after Your own heart. Give him or her a heart for what is right, pure, lovely, and good. Help me watch over my baby and bring up my child in a godly way. Help me be an example of Matthew 5:8, where You said, "Blessed are the pure in heart, for they shall see God" (NKJV).

Lord, bond us together as a family. Jesus, we invite You to be the head of our home and central to everything we do. Make us aware of Your presence in our lives on a daily basis. And bless our extended family as well.

If I have any ill feelings toward my parents, I pray that You will help me mend these relationships before my baby arrives, or use this baby in a special way to bring us back together. I want this baby to know his or her grandparents and receive their love as well. Bless us with an extended family.

Lord, I also pray that You develop my baby's heart just perfectly and make it beat in perfect rhythm for all the days of his or her life. Thank You, Lord, for this special gift.

In Jesus' name. Amen.

# Week 10

But the Helper, the Holy Spirit, whom the Father will send in My name, He will teach you all things, and bring to your remembrance all things that I said to you.

John 14:26 NKJV

At week 10, all your baby's vital organs have been formed and are beginning to work together, according to God's marvelous design. You're one-quarter of the way through your pregnancy.

What's going on at this point in your pregnancy is nothing short of astounding. Your baby's brain is generating 250,000 neurons every minute! Interestingly, the study of memory in neuroscience reveals two types of memory, which are performed in different regions of the brain:

1. Procedural memory, which is related to tasks and can be improved with repetition or practice. This type of memory is used when your baby learns that being snuggled in a certain way means he or she will soon be fed milk.
2. Declarative memory, which involves learning facts, such as telephone numbers. This type of memory is used when your baby learns to memorize and recognize your face and he or she responds to you more than to your friends.

And here's another significant finding: studies have shown that babies react more strongly to sounds they heard while still in their mother's womb than to new sounds introduced after birth.[1] This shows that your baby's memory is already at work!

This week, your baby officially progresses from being an embryo to a fetus, and congenital abnormalities are unlikely to develop after this week. Here's a tip: If you ever get tempted to worry about your baby's development, turn that energy into positive prayer instead. Here's a story from my experience.

## My Story

"Your baby could have Down syndrome," said the doctor.

I couldn't move, I couldn't blink, and I couldn't speak. How could this be happening?

"I'm going to refer you to a specialist." He said this like it was the next logical step, but to my mind, there was nothing logical about it.

How does a parent handle being told their child might have a condition they weren't expecting, which could mean extra challenges? I had to stop my mind from racing through all the what-ifs. I prayed constantly that week. It didn't matter what I was doing; I was praying and pleading with God for my unborn baby.

Finally, the day of our appointment with the specialist came. We were worried about the outcome, but we would keep and love our baby regardless. This specialist's ultrasound was amazing; we could see with perfect clarity our baby was on the move, wiggling and rolling around. The heartbeat was good, and all the limbs were the correct measurements for a baby that age. We were starting to feel reassured. Then the doctor came in.

He took one look and said, "There's the problem—Swiss cheese placenta!"

He went on to explain that this placenta works fine for the baby, but it does throw out abnormal protein levels into the blood, which explained why the tests came back positive.

The specialist said, "Your baby is fine. Everything is normal. Don't worry about a thing!"

I burst into tears. All I could say was, "Thank You, Lord. You've answered my prayers."

In hindsight, I see that this was a time when I grew closer to God. When you experience setbacks or stress during your pregnancy, lean on the Lord.

Lord, this week, I am feeling and thinking about:

What are You saying to me?

Something special I remember while I was pregnant:

Your dad's memory of my pregnancy:

This week, I release to God my cares and concerns about:

## A Mother's Prayer for Week 10

Dear Lord,

I pray for my baby's brain development. I pray that my baby will develop a healthy, intelligent brain. And because Your Word says, "Whatever you ask in My name, I will do" (John 14:13), I ask confidently, in faith. I also ask that You will bless my baby with an excellent memory. Lord, help me teach my baby to memorize Scriptures easily and quickly and to live out the principles that he or she learns.

Psalm 119:11 says, "Your word have I hidden in my heart, that I might not sin against You" (NKJV). I believe it is Your will to hide Your Word in our hearts, and I ask that for my child. I pray that Bible verses will come to his or her memory quickly in times of need. I thank You for Your promise of giving us peace, so I don't have to worry about something being wrong with my baby. I declare the power of Your Word and Your Holy Spirit to come to pass. May my baby's brain develop just as it should, and may my child be blessed with a high IQ, to be used for Your glory.

In Jesus' name I pray. Amen.

# Week 11

> Now as we have many parts in one body, and all the parts do not have the same function, in the same way we who are many are one body in Christ and individually members of one another. According to the grace given to us, we have different gifts.
>
> Romans 12:4–6

Don't feel bad if you need to reach out to someone to get perspective on your roller-coaster emotions. God made us to need one another. In fact, Romans 12 talks about how the different parts of our physical body depend on the other parts and compares this to the different members of the Body of Christ depending on one another. During the first trimester especially, changing hormones can take their toll on your energy and emotions. If you're feeling depressed, please find a trusted adviser, such as a Christian counselor or even a mom from your church who has experienced depression, to talk to and pray with. Don't try to struggle through your feelings on your own.

God's plans are amazing and wonderful, and this week, God's plans for your baby's development include tiny tooth buds growing under the gums. You probably won't see a tooth push through until your child is between four and twelve months old, but the start of your baby's teeth is there already.

In week eight, we talked about the hands and fingers, the feet and toes. This week, exquisitely small fingernail and toenail beds begin to develop. Facial development continues, and ears take their position. To accommodate all this development, the blood vessels in your placenta are increasing in order to meet the increasing nutritional needs of your baby.

## Your Baby's Sense of Smell

The latest research shows that babies can perceive odors from as early as 11 to 15 weeks. When you think of your sense of smell, what comes to mind?

Is it the sweet scent of roses, your grandmother's homemade cinnamon-apple pie, or a baby's skin after a warm bath? Pleasant thoughts may come to mind, but God also gave us this sense for our safety. The ability to smell a smoldering fire or detect toxic chemicals can save lives.

What's so amazing about an unborn baby's ability to smell is that, unlike previously thought, he or she doesn't need air or the ability to breathe in order to stimulate the olfactory organ. Now scientists tell us the amniotic fluid passes through the baby's mouth and nose, triggering the senses of taste and smell.[1]

With all the changes going on at this point, it's no wonder an expectant mom may feel a little overwhelmed on some days!

Lord, this week, I am feeling and thinking about:

_____

_____

_____

_____

_____

_____

_____

What are You saying to me?

_____

_____

_____

_____

_____

_____

_____

People I can reach out to if I need to share or to pray:

This week, I release to God my cares and concerns about:

## A Mother's Prayer for Week 11

Dear God,

I pray for my baby's teeth. You know how important it is to have good, strong teeth and a pleasant smile, and Your Word tells us that when we are concerned with something, You are concerned as well. I ask You to bless my child with good teeth. Help my baby's mouth to form just as it should and cause the teeth to fit perfectly. And, Lord, thank You for giving us the sense of smell. Please help my baby's perception of aromas develop just the way it should.

Thank You for all the amazing developments that are happening this week inside and outside my baby's body. When I feel tired or overwhelmed, help me remember that You are with me and You strengthen me. Let me experience Your peace with all the changes that are going on in my body, and peace in knowing that You love my baby and are guiding the development according to Your plans.

In Jesus' name. Amen.

# Week 12

Your baby is now practicing for when he or she will eat real food! Quite literally, your baby is flexing the digestive muscle, causing contraction movements. After birth, your child will use this skill to push food through his or her digestive tract.

Even though the digestive system is developing now, most doctors agree that newborns continue in this development after birth up to the first 13 weeks of life. Also noteworthy: new infants have not yet developed the probiotics that aid digestion. This may explain why some babies are colicky, crying from the discomfort of excess gas trapped in their intestines and bloating in their stomachs. I encourage you to pray for your baby's digestive system during this twelfth week in the womb and on throughout their infancy. Praying against allergies was also something I prayed for diligently and consistently while I was pregnant. I prayed that my baby wouldn't inherit allergies from me. I'm so glad we pray to a God who is real and who hears our prayers! To this day, our son and daughter do not have any allergies.

Some people might wonder if that was God's doing, and I believe it was. God's Word supports asking for what we need. John 14:13 says, "Whatever you ask in My name, I will do it so that the Father may be glorified in the Son." John 16:24 says, "Ask and you will receive, so that your joy may be complete." Just as we take delight in answering our children's requests, God wants to answer ours, so be encouraged to pray.

## A Heart of Compassion

Have you ever thought about how you would handle it if your child is "different"? For myself, having allergies so bad when I was a child made me different. I especially appreciated the people who were compassionate and sensitive to me. These are two Christlike traits to pray for your baby this week.

When I was pregnant, I asked God to give my baby a sensitive and compassionate heart. And you know what? He did. I first began to realize it when our son, Micah, was just a baby. He was an extremely happy baby and rarely cried. I remember being at the grocery store one afternoon, and there was a little one crying near us. Micah, who was probably four months old, looked at the baby and got tears in his eyes, and he started crying. It was really sweet, and he's continued to respond to others with sensitivity and compassion over the years. As a toddler, if he ever saw someone with pain or hurt in their eyes, he would ask me what was wrong with the person. He felt their pain.

Throughout the Gospels we see how Jesus showed compassion toward the sick and toward sinners (sparing the woman caught in adultery and dining with the cheating tax collector). Look at what was written by the prophet about Jesus: "The LORD has anointed Me to bring good news to the poor. He has sent Me to heal the brokenhearted, to proclaim liberty to the captives and freedom to the prisoners" (Isa. 61:1).

Pray that your baby will have those admirable traits too.

Lord, this week, I am feeling and thinking about:

_____

_____

_____

_____

_____

_____

What are You saying to me?

_____

_____

_____

_____

_____

_____

I can be a role model for my child in showing sensitivity and compassion to others by:

This week, I release to God my cares and concerns about:

## A Mother's Prayer for Week 12

Dear Lord,

This is a special week for my baby. It's the last week of the first trimester and the week in which his or her digestive system is beginning to develop. Lord, please help my baby develop a strong, healthy system that works in perfect order. I know that many people rely on digestive supplements and over-the-counter medicines to help them in this area, but I pray that my baby will not need anything like that.

Jesus, allergies can be life-threatening and bothersome. Please allow my baby to be free from any allergies whatsoever. You have the power to do that, and I ask this in Your name.

This week, I'd also pray for Your hand in giving my baby a sensitive and compassionate heart. Help my baby to see others in need and to love them like You do. Help my baby grow up to be a person who brings good news, heals broken hearts, and proclaims liberty and freedom to all. Give my child a Christlike attitude toward his family and everyone he meets.

In Jesus' name I pray. Amen.

Second Trimester

# Weeks 13–27

For it was You who created my inward parts;
You knit me together in my mother's womb.

Psalm 139:13

# Week 13

Let the words of my mouth and the meditation of my heart
Be acceptable in Your sight,
O LORD, my strength and my Redeemer.

Psalm 19:14 NKJV

What a fantastic feeling: you've made it to the second trimester! For most women, morning sickness and the risk of miscarrying are now in the past.

This week, your baby's vocal cords are developing! The Scriptures tell us that our tongue holds the power to speak love, peace, and life, or it can speak hatred, criticism, and death (see Prov. 18:21).

An 18-month-old child has a speaking vocabulary of 20 words, on average. Just six months later, the vocabulary has grown to 200 to 300 words. One year later, at three years of age, the average speaking vocabulary is 900 words. By the time a child is six and ready for first grade, the vocabulary is 2,600 words.[1]

One study estimates the average American adult has a vocabulary of 42,000 words.[2] And yet, the English language has hundreds of thousands of words. That's a lot of words to use for good or evil!

Some people, like my husband, Dan, use their words to earn a living. When we had been married for just two years, our lives were thrown into a tailspin the day Dan came home from work and could hardly talk.

"What's going on?" I asked him.

"I don't know," he squeaked out in a raspy whisper.

This went on for more than eight months—not good for someone who is a public speaker. We were in a real dilemma.

Finally, a specialist told us Dan had nodules on his vocal cords. Surgery was the only option to restore his voice—but it also might not be successful and he could completely lose his voice forever. In the car after the appointment with the specialist, we went over each scenario. Dan decided to go ahead with the surgery.

The hardest thing about this ordeal was that we wouldn't know whether the surgery was a success for 48 hours because he was not allowed to talk. We drove home in silence, each with our own thoughts and prayers. We tried to put fear out of our minds as we expected God to do great things through this situation.

Sunday morning, our alarm woke us up for church. Still groggy from sleep, out of habit I asked, "What time is it?"

"It's 9:00 a.m.," Dan announced in a totally normal voice—one I hadn't heard for eight months!

With tears in my eyes, I jumped on him and looked at his face. "You can talk! You can talk!" We were both so happy. We lay there and thanked God for giving Dan back his voice.

## Words Have Power

Words have the ability to lift up and encourage, or discourage and even bring spiritual death. Psalm 19:14 says, "Let the words of my mouth and the meditation of my heart be acceptable in Your sight, O Lord, my strength and my Redeemer" (NKJV).

It's not too early to pray that your child will reject negative words such as:

- "I hate myself" or "I hate you."
- "There is no reason to live."
- "I'm not good enough."
- "Nobody cares."

We need to help our children speak positive words by modeling positive speech ourselves, and now is the time to put it into practice and pray toward that end. When you speak a positive message and claim Scriptures through prayer, you release the power of the Holy Spirit to work on your behalf. Pray that your child will use this gift to speak truth and life into every circumstance.

Lord, this week, I am feeling and thinking about:

_____

_____

_____

_____

_____

_____

What are You saying to me?

_____

_____

_____

_____

_____

_____

The positive words I am speaking over my baby today:

This week, I release to God my cares and concerns about:

## A Mother's Prayer for Week 13

Dear Lord,

I praise You for the miracle of this baby I'm carrying. Truly, You are a great and wonderful God! I'm amazed at the exquisite detail You planned for Your creation. Thank You for caring for my unborn baby, as You said in so many verses.

I pray for my baby's vocal cord development—that his or her voice will develop properly. Help his or her mouth, throat, larynx, and windpipe to form as they should. And, Lord, I pray that my child will grow up to be a person who is known for speaking words of life. Help my child to speak only positive, encouraging, and uplifting words, and to avoid gossip, negativity, and criticism.

Help me, too, so that I can be a good role model for godly speech. Please help me when I'm having a hard day, when I'm tired, or when I'm angry, because I don't want to say things I'll regret later. Help me to hold my tongue. And when I do mess up, Lord, help me to ask for forgiveness quickly. Thank You, Lord, that we can call on You for help.

In Jesus' name. Amen.

> For you are all sons of God through faith in Christ Jesus. For as many of you as have been baptized into Christ have put on Christ.
>
> Galatians 3:26–27

This week, your baby's thyroid gland, which produces hormones and regulates metabolism, begins working. The roof of your baby's mouth is formed, and your baby displays a sucking reflex. And by this week, he or she has fully developed sex organs. What's even more amazing is that your baby also has the makings of becoming a parent.

If it's a girl, her ovaries are moving into place. If it's a boy, his prostate is forming now. One day, your child will have the ability to make you a grandparent—and it's already history in the making!

What will your baby inherit from you, and what will your grandchild and great-grandchild inherit from you?

It's remarkable what parents can pass on to their children. Everyone talks about a baby having his or her father's eyes, his or her mother's hair, or his or her grandma's long fingers that will surely play the piano someday. But a lot of us don't think about the fact that our child can also inherit our negative characteristics like a short temper, a pessimistic outlook, or even an unforgiving attitude, especially by our own words and actions. That's why I believe it's important to pray for your unborn baby's future character qualities. This week, pray that he or she will receive a legacy of love, joy, peace, patience, kindness, goodness, faith, gentleness, and self-control from both you and your husband (see Gal. 5:22–23).

Don't give in to negative thoughts such as, *I hope my child doesn't get Dad's bad temper or so-and-so's drinking problem*. Instead, claim the characteristics that Galatians 5:22–23 calls the fruit of the Spirit, which is the result of living a life filled with the Holy Spirit. A history of problems in your family tree does not mean it is your legacy or your children's legacy. Revelation 21:5 tells us that Jesus came to make all things new. Every individual who names Jesus Christ as their Lord and Savior has the right to put on the righteousness of God in Christ (see 2 Cor. 5:21). Colossians 1:12 says, "Giving thanks to the Father, who has enabled you to share in the saints' inheritance in the light." This is your child's legacy. Claim the promises in God's Word for yourself and for your children.

Lord, this week, I am feeling and thinking about:

_____

_____

_____

_____

_____

_____

What are You saying to me?

_____

_____

_____

_____

_____

_____

_____

The attitudes and characteristics I want to teach and become an example of for my baby:

_____

_____

_____

_____

_____

The characteristics I will ask Jesus to help me overcome so I don't become a negative example to my child (for example, anger, selfishness, unthankfulness, rudeness):

_____

_____

_____

_____

_____

This week, I release to God my cares and concerns about:

## A Mother's Prayer for Week 14

Dear Lord,

I pray for my child that he or she will exhibit the fruit of the Holy Spirit: love, joy, peace, patience, kindness, goodness, faith, gentleness, and self-control. Help me to be a role model of these. Lord, I want to live my life connected to You so that I bring Your Spirit into our home and into my child's life. Help me be the loving mother You want me to be.

And, Lord, I pray for the physical development of my baby. Please cause everything that is happening this week to develop properly.

Psalm 139:13 says, "You created my inmost being; you knit me together in my mother's womb" (NIV). I thank You for this encouraging Scripture. Please knit together—cause to develop properly—every part of my baby's being: body, soul, and spirit.

In Jesus' name. Amen.

# Week 15

Casting all your care on Him, because He cares about you.

1 Peter 5:7

This week, your baby's delicate, translucent skin continues to develop, and he or she has a layer of downy-fine hair covering the skin, which protects it before birth. And two tiny eyebrows appear above your baby's eyes. The eyelashes are growing too. Hair is beginning to grow on your baby's head now. It's only the temporary hair at this stage. Some babies are born bald, but most have hair by the time they're six months old. Will your child's hair be curly, wavy, or straight? Black, brown, red, blond, or a shade in between? It's fun to imagine what your baby will look like.

Human hair is controlled by more than one gene. It's not as simple as a child taking after the mother's or father's side. The unknown question is, which parent has the dominant version of the gene?

Every person carries two copies of every gene—one from the mom and one from the dad. Several different genes control the hair, each with two or more versions called alleles. The different versions can combine in unpredictable ways to produce a wide variety of appearances. Hair color is a result of interaction between several genes that control not only color but also how much pigment (darkness level) is deposited into the hair shaft. It's all very interesting.

Speaking of inheriting traits from parents and grandparents, genetic scientists tell us that skin color is probably the most complex of all physical traits. According to the latest estimates, there are about six genes that determine skin color, and since we have two copies of each gene (one each from mom and dad), there are 12 possible contributions to the skin color trait. This means that your baby can have from 0 to 12 genes that give varying dosages of color. Your baby randomly receives six genes from you and six from your husband. It's like a beautiful, complex puzzle created by God. And only He knows in advance what your baby's skin tone will look like.

Your baby's skin will do more than make him or her look beautiful. The skin is the body's largest organ, and it functions in four ways:

1. It helps regulate body temperature.
2. It protects the internal organs from physical and chemical injury.
3. It protects the body from invasion of microorganisms.
4. It synthesizes vitamin D, which is diffused into the blood vessels. (Infants and children who lack vitamin D can get a bone malady called rickets.)

As you pray this week, pray that your child will be content with the way God made him or her. First Timothy 6:6 says, "Godliness with contentment is a great gain."

Lord, this week, I am feeling and thinking about:

_____

_____

_____

_____

_____

_____

What are You saying to me?

_____

_____

_____

_____

_____

_____

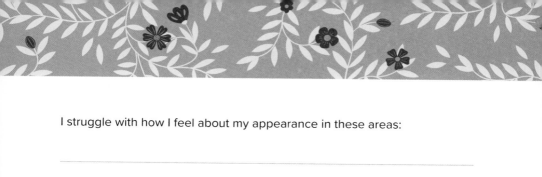

I struggle with how I feel about my appearance in these areas:

I can help my child be content with his or her appearance by:

This week, I release to God my cares and concerns about:

## A Mother's Prayer for Week 15

Dear Lord,

I pray for my baby's hair and skin. Thank You for the wonderful way You make us, with hair to beautify our appearance. I pray that as my child grows, he or she will be pleased with the type of hair You've given him or her. Help me instill healthy self-esteem in my child, so he or she grows up to be a happy person, content with the way he or she looks.

I pray for my baby's skin, that it will be healthy and perform the functions You've created it to do. Thank You for giving us beauty combined with protection in the organ that is our skin.

You are a wonderful, loving God. Your Word says that You even know the number of hairs on our head, and I know that means You are concerned with every detail of us. Thank You for caring and loving us so much. I praise You for my baby, growing inside me. I know that You love my baby and see my child even as he or she is yet unborn.

In Jesus' name. Amen.

# Week 16

For it was You who created my inward parts;
You knit me together in my mother's womb.

Psalm 139:13

If you could observe your baby's face right now, you'd see a variety of expressions. Yes, your baby's facial features and muscles are developed enough for him or her to frown, smirk, and grin. It would be cute if your baby was frowning when he or she heard you say you don't feel well and grinning when he or she thought about coming out and meeting you, but I don't think that's the case. But at this point, your baby's face is definitely sensitive, even to a light touch.

Your baby continues to grow and is now about three ounces and between four and five inches long. No wonder you're hungry!

If you're having a girl, here's a mind-boggling fact: this week, millions of eggs are forming in her ovaries. God has already planned your future grandchildren!

My deepest desire and prayer for my children is that they will always follow after God, and that He will be the One to write the story of their lives. I pray that they will know God and make Him known, like the Bible says.

It's never too soon to pray about future events. Your words have power; you can speak life through the act of blessing your unborn child and then continuing to speak that blessing as he or she grows up. You can say things to your baby such as, "May you grow up to be a man after God's own heart" or "May you be a woman who loves the Lord your God with all your heart, soul, mind, and strength."

An equally significant way to affect your child's destiny is to pray God's Word over your baby as a way of affirming God's care and His faithfulness to His promises. Choose a Scripture verse or passage you will use as a special daily prayer for your unborn child. For example: "I pray that 'you may live a life worthy of the Lord and please him in every way'" (Col.

1:10 NIV). It's okay to paraphrase Scripture to personalize it. Here is an example from Proverbs 31 for a daughter: "I pray that you will speak with wisdom, and that faithful instruction will be on your tongue. I pray that you will watch over the affairs of your household, that your children will arise and call you blessed, that your husband will do the same, and he will praise you" (vv. 26–28, paraphrased).

There are so many biblical prayers and blessings for you to search out and choose for your child. If you'd like to read more examples, take a look at the apostle Paul's beginning words in each of his letters to the Galatians, the Ephesians, the Philippians, and the Colossians. Or check out the spiritual armor passage in Ephesians 6, beginning with verse 10. And don't forget scriptural blessings like the one found in Jude 24–25.

Lord, this week, I am feeling and thinking about:

What are You saying to me?

Scriptures I want to pray over my baby:

_____

_____

_____

_____

_____

_____

_____

_____

_____

_____

_____

_____

_____

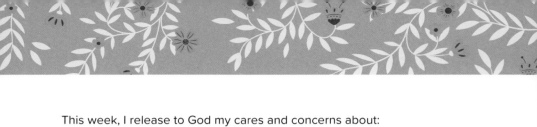

This week, I release to God my cares and concerns about:

_____

_____

_____

_____

_____

_____

_____

_____

_____

_____

_____

_____

_____

## A Mother's Prayer for Week 16

Dear Lord,

I pray for my baby's growth. As his or her face continues to develop, please cause everything to come together to form a beautiful child.

If I'm having a girl, I pray for her ovaries and eggs that will give her children someday. Lord, Your plans are so awesome. Your Word says that children are an inheritance from the Lord, and I pray that my daughter will have the blessing of being a mother one day. And, God, I pray for my daughter's future husband, that You will bring a good, kind, loving, wise man into her life, and most of all, that he will be a man of God who loves You and follows Your Word.

If I'm having a boy, I pray for my son's future wife. Bless her and bring her and my son together in Your timing. I pray that she will be a woman who loves my son and is a good and faithful wife, but most of all, that she is a woman of God who loves You and follows Your Word. Lord, You said that You delight in giving us the desires of our heart, so I ask that I will have a special, loving relationship with the mates of my children, that we will all get along and enjoy one another's company. I also ask for the blessing of being an integral part of my grandchildren's lives to help them, to pass on wisdom, and to be a blessing to them.

In Jesus' name. Amen.

# Week 17

Your baby is gaining body fat this week, plumping up, and will continue to do so until he or she is born. This is a good thing, as long as your baby is adding the normal layers of fat that are necessary for keeping the baby warm after his or her entrance into the world. But in our modern culture, too often unborn babies are forced into obesity by mothers who eat double and triple the calories they need to support their pregnancy. An overweight newborn is disadvantaged from the get-go, because he or she is at risk for acquiring obesity-related health problems.[1]

On the opposite end, we live in a society that puts a tremendous amount of value on being slim and attractive, so some moms-to-be don't eat enough while they are pregnant. Overall, many people have an issue with self-image and body weight. I was affected by this myself.

Growing up in Hawaii, I spent a lot of time enjoying the outdoors, and my family led an active lifestyle. But then I went away to college in California, and so many things changed. Like a lot of college girls, I gained more than the "freshman 15"; I gained the "freshman 40"—and I'm only 5'2", so that was a lot of extra weight for me.

When I returned home after a year, someone dear to me looked at me and said, "What the heck happened to you?" That didn't make me feel very good! So I decided right then and there to make a life change.

I became involved in fitness training and lost 42 pounds in six months. I loved fitness training so much that I went on to become a certified fitness trainer and nutrition expert.

As you can imagine, the last thing in the world I wanted to do when I became pregnant was to gain a lot of extra weight and go back to how

I was while in college. So weight gain and health are both important issues for me. I studied and worked hard to gain only a healthy amount of weight and to have a healthy pregnancy and healthy baby.

One thing we want for our children is for them to have a healthy self-image and to be happy with their body. We don't want them to compare themselves to anyone, especially celebrities or anorexic models. We want them to be healthy, to feel good about themselves, and to know that their parents and God love them very much just as they are.

This week, let's work on honoring God with our bodies. Pray that your unborn baby will gain a healthy amount of body fat and have a healthy self-image. And then for the future, pray that your baby will develop inner beauty that is lasting. It's never too soon to pray for your child's self-esteem and body image. Our children definitely need our prayer support. As 1 Peter 3:3–4 says, "Your beauty . . . should consist of what is inside the heart with the imperishable quality of a gentle and quiet spirit, which is very valuable in God's eyes."

Lord, this week, I am feeling and thinking about:

_____

_____

_____

_____

_____

_____

What are You saying to me?

_____

_____

_____

_____

_____

_____

How I can help my child understand that inner beauty is the most important type of beauty:

_____

_____

_____

_____

_____

_____

_____

_____

_____

_____

_____

_____

_____

This week, I release to God my cares and concerns about:

## A Mother's Prayer for Week 17

Dear Lord,

As my baby continues to grow, I pray that he or she will gain the right amount of weight, including a healthy amount of body fat. Please help me to eat in a healthy way and exercise on a regular basis so I don't put my baby in jeopardy of having diabetes or other obesity-related health issues. Give me the strength to avoid junk foods and excessive sugar and fat.

Lord, also help me to concentrate on good health and not become obsessed with body weight and body image. I know my self-worth comes from You and not from the way I look. Please help me to remember that, and help me pass on to my child only good attitudes about his or her appearance and weight. Protect my child from eating disorders and a poor self-image.

Empower us, as a family, to live a healthy lifestyle. Empower us to be good testimonies of Your love, forgiveness, and life-changing power. I pray that we would shine from an inner glow of Your Holy Spirit and that it would attract people to You.

And, Father God, please continue to bless and guide my baby's development. I thank You for Your love and protection.

In Jesus' name. Amen.

# Week 18

> So God created man in His own image;
> He created him in the image of God;
> He created them male and female.
>
> Genesis 1:27

If you're having a girl, her uterus and fallopian tubes are developed by the end of this week. And if you're having a boy, his prostate and genitals continue to develop.

What a marvelous message from God in the verse above, that He designed us to be in His own image, able to communicate with Him, and to be male or female—both His design!

During my pregnancies and even continuing on now, I pray for my son and daughter to celebrate how God made them, and yet to exercise sexual purity. It's a great challenge for our young people to stay sexually pure until marriage. Our children are bombarded with sexual messages, and I pray for my children to hold on to God's Word and have the strength to say no to temptation. It might not be popular, but following God's way of abstinence saves a lot of heartache and, oftentimes, disaster. I'm sure we all know young men and women who have been hurt by becoming sexually active before marriage.

I was one of those teens. I learned the hard way, and now I pray that my children do not engage in premarital sex. First Peter 2:11 says to "abstain from fleshly desires that war against you."

When I was 12, someone very close to me got pregnant at 15. I remember feeling stunned when I found out; I just couldn't believe it. As a result, she had to drop out of high school to try to raise her child.

She had a friend who offered to help her get an abortion. And her family knew people who would adopt the baby, if that's what she chose. Thank God she had wonderful Christian parents and friends who didn't judge her but reached out in compassion to help her instead. The end of this story is a happy one. Her circle of support helped her to raise a wonderful daughter and send her to a Christian school, where she became the valedictorian of her graduating class. I am proud to say this young mother was my sister.

As parents, we want and hope for the best for our children. We teach them and pray that they will overcome temptation and wait until they get married to have sexual relations. So this week, not judging or condemning anyone, pray for your children to highly value sexual purity and follow God's way.

Lord, this week, I am feeling and thinking about:

_____

_____

_____

_____

_____

_____

What are You saying to me?

_____

_____

_____

_____

_____

_____

How I will encourage my son or daughter toward sexual purity and abstaining from sex until marriage:

This week, I release to God my cares and concerns about:

## A Mother's Prayer for Week 18

Dear Lord,

I pray for the sexual development that's going on in my baby's body. I thank You that You made us so wonderfully, and I pray that my baby's body and hormones will develop properly, just as You designed.

And, Lord, I pray for sexual purity for my child. Help me to teach my child to follow Your ways, and give me wisdom to answer tough questions. Help me keep watch over my child and protect him or her, as a godly parent should. Make my child strong against temptation and the pull of the world. I pray that he or she will not sacrifice godly principles for popularity. Instill Scriptures in my child's heart so that he or she does not sin against You, as Psalm 119:11 says. Protect my family and keep us under the shelter of Your Holy Spirit.

In Jesus' name. Amen.

# Week 19

The one who lives under the protection of the Most High
dwells in the shadow of the Almighty.
I will say to the Lord, "My refuge and my fortress,
my God, in whom I trust."

Psalm 91:1–2

You might get some clues about your baby's personality this week. Do you have a content, peaceful child who smiles, yawns, and has a long, leisurely stretch? Or do you have a real go-getter, doing flips and somersaults? Get ready, because your baby is capable of performing a lot of action this week and from this point on. I think it's got to be one of the most awesome experiences to feel a growing baby inside of you, moving.

I remember the first time I felt "something." It can be like you're not sure if it's the baby or just gas. But then you feel it again—and you know, someone else is growing inside of you.

Up to this week, your baby has had his or her legs curled and tucked under, but now he or she has straightened them out. You might feel some dancing or gymnastics going on in there! And did you know that on ultrasound images, they've even seen babies open their mouth and stick out their tongue?

Take a look at all the things your baby can do when he or she is not sleeping:

- smile and frown
- suck and swallow
- hiccup
- breathe
- yawn
- stretch
- rotate

- lift his or her head
- flip
- somersault
- open his or her mouth and stick out his or her tongue

Yes, you've got a dynamic person with his or her own unique personality already being acted out inside of you.

Who knows what cute signature moves your baby may be making now, while he or she is growing inside you? Well, don't worry; soon you'll get to see those moves every day, because you're almost halfway to your delivery date. This week, pray not only for your baby's growth, but also for his or her personality and for the joy of the Lord to always be with your child. Whether you have a thoughtful, quiet introvert or a rambunctious extrovert, I think that as mothers and fathers, what we want most is for our children to know the love of God and to have His joy surround them no matter what this world brings their way. Here are some Scriptures to focus your mind on the joy of the Lord and His desires for us:

> Take delight in the LORD,
>     and he will give you the desires of your heart. (Ps. 37:4 NIV)

> Happy are the people whose God is Yahweh. (Ps. 144:15)

I pray that God, the source of hope, will fill you completely with joy and peace because you trust in Him. Then you will overflow with confident hope through the power of the Holy Spirit. (Rom. 15:13 NLT)

Lord, this week, I am feeling and thinking about:

_____

_____

_____

_____

_____

_____

_____

What are You saying to me?

_____

_____

_____

_____

_____

_____

_____

Lord, it says in Your Word that we can be filled with joy and peace from Your Spirit. I want my child to be filled with happiness and joy as well. Here is my prayer for my child:

This week, I release to God my cares and concerns about:

## A Mother's Prayer for Week 19

Dear Lord,

I praise You for this wonderful life growing inside of me. I pray that my baby will continue to grow properly and be 100 percent healthy. Cause all the parts of the body to grow right and be strong. And, Lord, I pray that my child will have a happy heart and joyful spirit. Give him or her a personality that draws others to want to be friends.

Lord, please make all my test results accurate, with a good outcome. Give the doctor or midwife wisdom. If anything is amiss at this point, heal my baby and make him or her totally and completely perfect, in Jesus' name. I stand on the Holy Bible that promises us that God heals ALL diseases. You are our Creator and Healer, Lord God, and I claim perfect health for my baby.

God, You are awesome, and I thank You for the miracle of this baby growing inside of me. Please help this entire pregnancy to go smoothly, and help me to enjoy this amazing time in my life. This truly is a gift from You, and I praise You for it. Thank You, Lord.

In Jesus' name. Amen.

# Week 20

Rejoice in hope; be patient in affliction; be persistent in prayer.

Romans 12:12

Good news! Week 20 is the official halfway point on the 40-week pregnancy calendar. It feels great to know that approximately half of your pregnancy is behind you!

The main event in your baby's development this week is the velvety-soft skin. It is separating into the four layers of the epidermis, and the skin for the palms of the hands and the bottoms of the feet is forming as well.

Remarkably, a protective layer of creamy white moisturizer, called the vernix, covers your baby's skin this week while it's developing.[1] This is no cheap drugstore product—this natural emollient performs multiple functions, such as the following:

- It protects your baby's skin from scratches.
- It contains the antioxidants vitamin E and melanin to help the skin cope with the baby's entry into air at birth.
- It has anti-infective properties to protect from bacterial invasion.
- It hydrates the skin.
- It may help regulate the temperature of the skin.

I was thinking about this extra-fancy moisturizer that protects the unborn baby, and it made me think about how good God is to watch out for every need we have. If God made your baby's oil glands to produce vernix, don't you think He cares about watching over your baby's health? Absolutely.

As simple as it may sound, prayer is the best way to connect with God about everything. God said He would work on your behalf when you pray and seek Him.

But too often we forget about having a deep relationship with the Lord through prayer, which will fill our hearts with peace and joy, the true gifts that our hearts desire. Instead, we worry. We talk to our friends, but we don't pray. And it's like God is saying, "I'd love to give you these important gifts that will make your life go a lot better, but you have to spend some time with Me." There is a great quote, often attributed to the great American evangelist Billy Graham, that reminds us, "Heaven is full of answers to prayers for which no one ever bothered to ask."[2] I, for one, don't want to be guilty of not seeking the Lord, spending time with Him, or asking Him for everything my children need, because I know He will always provide for us according to His perfect will.

Here are a few verses to encourage you to continue to pray for what you and your baby need:

> The LORD is near to all who call on him,
> to all who call on him in truth. (Ps. 145:18 ESV)

You will call to Me and come and pray to Me, and I will listen to you. (Jer. 29:12)

Be joyful in hope, patient in affliction, faithful in prayer. (Rom. 12:12 NIV)

Do not be anxious about anything, but in everything by prayer and supplication with thanksgiving let your requests be made known to God. (Phil. 4:6 ESV)

Lord, this week, I am feeling and thinking about:

_____

_____

_____

_____

_____

_____

What are You saying to me?

_____

_____

_____

_____

_____

_____

How my expectations have increased and/or changed since the beginning of my pregnancy:

_____

_____

_____

_____

_____

_____

_____

_____

_____

_____

_____

_____

This week, I release to God my cares and concerns about:

## A Mother's Prayer for Week 20

Dear Lord,

I thank You for hearing and answering my prayers. Your Word tells us that You are touched by our feelings and that You care for us. And, Jesus, You showed how much You loved the little children when You took them in Your arms and blessed them. So this week, I thank You that I've made it to the halfway point on the pregnancy calendar, and I pray for my baby's continued growth and development.

It is so awesome the way You designed pregnancy to take care of a baby's needs. I pray for my baby's skin as it is growing the four layers this week. Help the moisturizing vernix to be produced and do its job. Protect my baby's skin from scratches, dehydration, and infection. When my baby is born, protect the skin from any harm.

Protect my baby, both physically and spiritually. Keep my child safe in Your loving arms.

In Jesus' name. Amen.

# Week 21

My soul, praise Yahweh,
and all that is within me, praise His holy name.
My soul, praise the LORD,
and do not forget all His benefits.

Psalm 103:1–2

The big news this week is that your baby's bone marrow—that flexible tissue inside the bones—is developed enough to produce blood cells. All blood cells are produced in the bone marrow, and most of a child's bones produce blood, which carries nutrients to every part of the body and then takes away the waste again.

It's important to have strong bones, both while growing up and while growing older. I grew up in a home where several people in the family had an allergy to dairy products, so we never had cow's milk in the house. To make sure we got enough calcium, every morning my father stirred calcium powder into our oatmeal, along with some honey. I also grew up drinking goat's milk, almond milk, or rice milk to add calcium to my diet.

The National Institutes of Health says that 99 percent of our body's total calcium is stored in our bones and teeth. When you're pregnant or breastfeeding, you need between 1,000 and 1,300 mg of calcium each day, depending on your age.[1] Check with your doctor about taking supplements that contain calcium along with magnesium and vitamin D to aid with calcium absorption; in addition, other good sources of calcium are low-fat yogurt, cheddar cheese, milk, cottage cheese, kale, and broccoli.

Because I'm a personal trainer, women have often asked me if it's okay to lift weights or do weight-bearing exercises during pregnancy. The answer is yes, as long as you lift the proper amount of weight for your fitness level and for your stage of pregnancy, and in the correct way. Exercising with weights benefits you in five ways:

1. Helps strengthen your bones and muscles
2. Improves your metabolism
3. Boosts your energy
4. Supports sound sleep
5. Helps keep you from gaining an unhealthy amount of excess weight, which is a concern during pregnancy

Try to do your best to maintain a workout schedule. During the first trimester, I had days of extreme tiredness and an upset stomach—which is normal due to hormonal changes—so I gave myself some grace on those days and didn't work out or just did a stretching routine. In my second trimester, I was able to keep a regular workout schedule. This included both weight-bearing exercises for strength, toning, and metabolism boosting, and aerobic exercises for endurance. In addition, stretching routines helped to keep my bones and muscles flexible and helped prevent injury.

Lord, this week, I am feeling and thinking about:

_____

_____

_____

_____

_____

_____

What are You saying to me?

_____

_____

_____

_____

_____

_____

With my energy level and ability right now, I can exercise by:

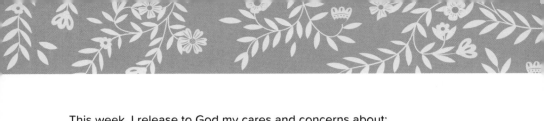

This week, I release to God my cares and concerns about:

_____

_____

_____

_____

_____

_____

_____

_____

_____

_____

_____

_____

_____

## A Mother's Prayer for Week 21

Dear Lord,

I pray for my baby's bones that are developing this week so they can produce life-giving blood cells. I ask You for bone marrow that is 100 percent healthy. I ask for the correct amount of red and white blood cells and platelets.

Lord, You promised to hear and answer our prayers. I claim the promise in Psalm 105:8: "He remembers His covenant forever, the promise He ordained for a thousand generations." You don't forget Your promises, and I thank You for that. You can do all things. You are the Creator of life. My hope is not dependent on myself or other people; You are my source of strength.

Lord, please give me the strength to eat healthy and to exercise. I know that proper exercise will benefit my unborn baby. Everything I eat, drink, and breathe goes into my baby, so please bless me with endurance and the strength to make the best choices.

And, Lord, I pray that my baby will be happy. Give him or her a heart filled with the joy of being alive. May my child find gladness in everyday things like a beautiful sunset, a cute puppy or kitten, a good book, or a dear friend. Give us many happy memories together.

In Jesus' name I pray. Amen.

# Week 22

How sweet Your word is to my taste—
sweeter than honey to my mouth.
I gain understanding from Your precepts.

Psalm 119:103–104

Good things are happening this week. Due to maturing brain cells and nerve endings, your baby's sense of touch becomes even more sensitive. The first area to experience more sensitivity is in the cheek, which may explain why your baby starts sucking his or her thumb in the womb. Ultrasound has discovered babies stroking their faces and feeling other parts of their bodies too, already exploring how they are made. Scientists estimate that by week 22, nearly every part of a baby's body perceives warmth, cold, pressure, and pain.

Also this week, your baby develops taste buds. The latest medical research tells us the taste buds are formed between weeks 9 and 15, so they are likely fully developed by this point. You might wonder if that really means anything now, before your son or daughter is born. The answer is yes, it does. The amniotic fluid surrounding your baby picks up flavors from your food, especially pungent flavors like curry, cumin, garlic, onion, and other spicy foods. If you love garlic or hot sauce, perhaps it is because your mother ate spicy food when she was pregnant with you. Research tells us that unborn babies swallow more in response to sweet tastes and swallow less in response to bitter and sour tastes.

Babies have a definite sense of taste at birth. Newborns demonstrate having opinions and preferences.[1]

## Praying for Your Baby's Happiness

The Bible uses a metaphor of taste to tell us how to be happy. Psalm 34:8 says, "Taste and see that the LORD is good. How happy is the man who takes refuge in Him!" This is a word picture inviting people to the Lord in order to experience happiness. It's interesting that the writer didn't say, "Taste and see if you like it." Instead, he said taste to see, or taste to discover, that the Lord is good. In other words, everyone who tries the Lord finds that He is good! A life with God is a life with true joy and happiness, because *God is good.*

It's odd now when I look back at the time before I was living for Jesus. I thought I was happy, but in reality, I was just going along on my own, and so much was missing that I didn't even know about. The awesome thing about being a Christian is that we have Jesus as our best friend. We're never alone. Through the good times and the bad, He is always with us. I fully realized this during my first year with our son, Micah.

This week, pray for your child's future and to receive the true happiness that only the Lord can give him or her.

Lord, this week, I am feeling and thinking about:

_____

_____

_____

_____

_____

_____

What are You saying to me?

_____

_____

_____

_____

_____

_____

God made so many flavors and foods, and right now I'm craving:

This week, I release to God my cares and concerns about:

## A Mother's Prayer for Week 22

Dear Lord,

Thank You for this week. The time is getting near, and I will soon get to see my newborn baby. I am so excited. Lord, help me to read Your Word to my baby, for I know that it is like honey in his or her mouth. I pray for health and true joy for my child. There is no greater joy for a mother than to see her children walking in the way of the Lord, as 3 John 4 says.

Give my child true happiness, not through wealth and riches, but from knowing You as his or her personal Savior. Help me teach my child to read and memorize Your Word and to have a hunger for the Word of Life.

Thank You, Lord, for this beautiful baby growing inside of me.

In Jesus' name. Amen.

# Week 23

Then the LORD God formed the man out of the dust from the ground and breathed the breath of life into his nostrils, and the man became a living being.

Genesis 2:7

Your baby's lungs are making huge progress this week, with blood vessels expanding and preparing your child to breathe after birth. Your baby makes breathing movements now, but he or she is just practicing. You still provide oxygen for your son or daughter through the placenta and umbilical cord. A baby's lungs are completely collapsed before birth, but his or her first breath inflates the lungs and opens up the small air sacs called alveoli, which transfer oxygen to the blood.

Biologists are intrigued by the question, What makes a baby start to breathe on his or her own? They think it's a combination of physical stimuli including cold, touch, temperature, and oxygen supply; the absence of a protein in the uterus that prohibits breathing; and the baby's own lung maturation. Study is ongoing. I like to think that an angel whispers in the baby's ear and tells him or her it's time to breathe. But either way, it's a wonderful miracle. Your baby's lungs might also provide a clue as to when you go into labor. A study conducted at UT Southwestern Medical Center in Dallas found evidence that a protein in the unborn baby's lungs could signal it's time to start the birth process.[1]

Although some babies can be born at week 23 and survive, it's better to have more time for lung development and for the other major organs to mature as well. Even so, this week is a milestone.

When our son, Micah, was born, the umbilical cord was wrapped around his neck—twice. The doctors think he aspirated, which may have caused "streaking" in his lungs. For his first two weeks, I carried him and his little oxygen tank around the house. I had him in a little Moses basket in one hand and the tank in the other. Nurses came to check on him almost every other day, and they all said that he just needed a little help with his breathing—something that was not uncommon in Denver, the Mile High City, with 17 percent less oxygen in its thin air.

I sat and prayed over him every day, that God would make his lungs stronger and that he would not need the oxygen tank anymore. I claimed the promise in Psalm 34:17: "The righteous cry out, and the LORD hears, and delivers them from all their troubles."

Finally, we went to his two-week checkup, and the doctor said, "Why is he on this? He's perfectly fine."

God answered our prayers! We were ecstatic!

God is our oxygen. He is our Breath of Life. Without Him, we cannot live. Genesis 2:7 tells us that God formed man and breathed into his nostrils, and the man became a living being. That is amazing to me. When your new one enters this world, you wait to hear your baby's cry. Every mother waits to hear the sound of her child's voice for confirmation that breath and life have occurred.

This week, pray for your baby's lungs as you remember the Giver of every breath.

Lord, this week, I am feeling and thinking about:

_____

_____

_____

_____

_____

_____

_____

What are You saying to me?

_____

_____

_____

_____

_____

_____

_____

As I read the following passages, I will consider the Holy Spirit's work in me, so I can "breathe" in a spiritually hostile environment: Ezekiel 36:27; Romans 8:9–18.

What helps my "spiritual lungs" work:

This week, I release to God my cares and concerns about:

## A Mother's Prayer for Week 23

Dear Lord,

I thank You for breathing the breath of life into my baby. You are amazing, God, and I acknowledge Your greatness and praise You.

Lord, please help my baby's lungs to continue to grow and develop and to form perfectly. Help me carry the baby to full term so the lungs and other organs have time to mature. Give my baby strong and healthy lungs, and strength and health in every way.

Lord, let us all use the breath You have given us to express gratitude and praise to You. And let us use the breath You've given us to pass on Your love to others. Help me to be a good role model for my family, and help me to be an expression of Your Holy Spirit. Thank You, Lord.

In Jesus' name I pray. Amen.

# Week 24

Look carefully then how you walk, not as unwise but as wise.

Ephesians 5:15 ESV

Scientists who study otolaryngology (the medical specialty concerned with the ear, nose, and throat) tell us the basic structure of the inner ear is present in unborn babies at 24 weeks. This means your baby can now hear and detect direction of motion, such as moving forward to backward, side to side, and up and down.

At this point, there's still enough room for your baby to turn upside down and back again—and he or she can tell which way is which. Some people have an extraordinary sense of direction, and they rarely get lost. You may know someone like that.

Because the inner ear is located close to the center of the skull, it is one of the best-protected sensory systems we have. It seems that God made it a priority to safeguard our hearing and balance.

One of the things that's important for us and our children is to have a good sense of balance when it comes to life management. Years ago, I became a certified personal trainer and nutrition counselor specializing in training for women. Many of my clients have been moms or moms-to-be. I love helping women improve their physical fitness, because it's important to take care of the body God has blessed us with. One of the ways we can glorify God in our body is by respecting it and taking proper care of it.

If you aren't really happy with your body, I want to encourage you to put a stop to any derogatory thoughts. Don't look in the mirror and say hateful things about your body. Instead, think about the positive progress you're going to make, and give yourself the respect that a vessel designed by God deserves. God made your body to be a perfect habitat to nurture, grow, and birth your baby, and that is a beautiful miracle.

If you are someone who tends to go overboard with fitness one way or another, now is the time to bring it back into balance. We don't want to neglect other areas of our life, or other important things like studying God's Word, spending time in prayer, and worshiping God with other believers.

Any type of obsession is out-of-balance behavior and eventually will cause harm. This week, pray for balance—for you and your baby!

## A Heart of Generosity

Another part of a balanced life is caring for others. There is great joy when we give to others, so I also want my children to learn about generosity at an early age. My grandma is one of the most generous people I know. When I was young, she brought us suitcases of gifts from Chicago all the way to Hawaii. Anything we asked for she would find and tuck away until her next trip. She barely brought anything in her bags for herself—it was always about us kids. And fortunately, she was able to visit three or four times a year.

Grandma treated each of her grandchildren the same, showering them with love by giving, and she did the same for her "adopted" grandchildren and others she met along life's way. She also gave to charities, and even later, when money was short for her, she never stopped giving to charities or to our family. Through her generosity, Grandma made a lasting impression on me, and I want to be this kind of role model so my children will grow up to be giving people, balanced in body and mind but also in service to others.

Lord, this week, I am feeling and thinking about:

_____

_____

_____

_____

_____

_____

What are You saying to me?

_____

_____

_____

_____

_____

_____

_____

What a balanced life looks like to me on a daily basis:

Where I need to grow in this area:

This week, I release to God my cares and concerns about:

## A Mother's Prayer for Week 24

Dear Lord,

It's amazing how You think of everything. You've placed each part where it should be. I pray for good hearing and a good sense of direction for my baby. Please keep my baby's ears safe and help him or her not to get earaches, as many young children do.

Lord, please give my baby a good sense of balance in life. Let him or her know what is important and yet not go overboard or be obsessive. Give my child the wisdom to know when to work, when to rest, and when to play. Let him or her know that with a balanced Christian life, following Your ways, there is a time for everything.

Thank You, Lord, for this gift of life. Please also help me to balance my own life according to Your will. Help me to know when to rest and just leave the undone housework alone. Help me to know when to say no to requests from other people. Help me take time to pray and meditate on Your Word. Let me be a good role model of living a balanced Christian life.

And, Jesus, please help me teach my children to be generous. It's hard sometimes in this society we live in, but You showed us examples all throughout the Bible of how we should give to others. Help me to be a good example.

In Jesus' name. Amen.

# Week 25

The LORD your God has blessed you in all the work of your hands.

Deuteronomy 2:7

Your baby's hands are now fully formed: 10 exquisite fingers, complete with miniature fingernails and even fingerprints. The pattern of loops, whorls, and arches your baby has on those fingers is his or her permanent, unique pattern.

Interestingly, about 1,750 years before the birth of Christ, Babylonians used fingerprints to sign their clay tablets. Even then, they knew people had individual patterns to the ridges on their fingers.

For me, the fingers and hands are some of the most important parts of my baby's body. You may remember that Helen Keller, a brilliant woman who was blind, deaf, and mute, learned to read, "hear," and "speak" by using the tips of her fingers in the palm of another person's hand, and vice versa.

One of my favorite memories of our son when he was a little boy is when he'd come and pet my face with his sticky little hands. He touched my cheeks and hair and said, "I love you, Mama." My heart just melted every time. I'd think, *I don't deserve such a wonderful little boy.* When I was still pregnant with him, I prayed diligently that he would always use his hands to help others and never use them to hurt anyone. And now that he has a little sister, I can see that God heard my prayers. To this day, Micah has never hit or hurt his sister. He'll walk up to her, touch her cheeks, and give her a kiss. I believe he will use his hands to protect her when they get older and that he will never harm her.

I encourage you, too, to pray for how your baby will use his or her hands. If your baby already has a brother or sister or may have one in the future, pray for their relationship. As a parent, you have the authority to stand for your children in prayer.

I like to use Scripture in my prayers, because Hebrews 4:12 says the Word of God is "living and effective," which means that when we pray using the Word of God, we're taking part in something that is alive! And it's effective, meaning it works. God's power is released when we pray.

Take hold of faith and proclaim peace and joy in your household, in Jesus' name.

Lord, this week, I am feeling and thinking about:

_____

_____

_____

_____

_____

_____

What are You saying to me?

_____

_____

_____

_____

_____

_____

My prayer for peace and friendship between my child and his or her (maybe future) siblings:

The people and things I can't wait for my child to experience through his or her sense of touch:

This week, I release to God my cares and concerns about:

## A Mother's Prayer for Week 25

Dear Lord,

Thank You for creating each of us as unique individuals, including our own unique fingerprints. I pray for my baby's hands and fingers. Lord, help my child use his or her hands only for good and never for harm. Help my child to be kind and gentle. Help him or her to use whatever talents You may give him or her, whether it's music, writing, sports, or whatever, to be a blessing to others and to You.

As it says in the Psalms, may my baby praise You with his or her hands by lifting them to You during times of worship. And, Lord, I claim Deuteronomy 2:7, which says, "The Lord your God has blessed you in all the work of your hands."

Lord, I also pray for my child's siblings. Help all our children to get along with one another and grow up to be close friends. I pray they will look out for each other and use their hands only for good.

In Jesus' name. Amen.

# Week 26

> I pray that the eyes of your heart may be enlightened in order that you may know the hope to which he has called you, the riches of his glorious inheritance in his holy people.
>
> Ephesians 1:18 NIV

Can your baby see inside your womb?

Yes! At about week 26 to 28, depending on your individual baby's growth, your baby will open his or her eyes and see for the very first time.

Vision is the last sense to mature. Up until now, a baby's eyes are sealed shut while the retinas develop, but during weeks 26 to 28, your baby will open his or her eyes. Babies even blink their eyelids.

What's more, doctors have detected as early as week 26 that a set of twins will open their eyes, blink, look at one another, reach out, and touch one another's faces—and then hold hands. How sweet is that!

Remember the Old Testament account of the twins Esau and Jacob being born (see Gen. 25:19–26)? As you may recall, Rebekah could not conceive, so her husband, Isaac, prayed to the Lord on her behalf, and she became pregnant—an excellent example of intercessory prayer. Back then, there were no ultrasound machines to detect twins, so when Rebekah felt some strange action going on, she went to the Lord and inquired, "Why is this happening to me?"

The Lord basically said, "You have twins who are engaging in sibling rivalry. Your two sons will grow up to become the fathers of two nations."

As they were born, the second son, Jacob, came out holding on to his brother Esau's heel, as if to say, "Hey, I've got you, and I'm ready to compete with you." Undoubtedly, Rebekah's twins could see one another before they were born.

Just as it's not totally silent inside your womb, neither is it totally dark. A small amount of light filters through if you're out in the sun or under bright lights. Medical science has confirmed that babies can see during this time in your pregnancy, and I think that's fantastic.

Pray for your baby's eyesight this week, but pray for his or her spiritual sight as well. We see or perceive God not with our physical eyes but with the eyes of our heart. That's a beautiful metaphor that comes from Ephesians 1:18. Look up Scripture this week as your model for praying for your baby's spiritual sight.

Lord, this week, I am feeling and thinking about:

_____

_____

_____

_____

_____

_____

What are You saying to me?

_____

_____

_____

_____

_____

_____

_____

A time when God opened my eyes and gave me spiritual vision:

This week, I release to God my cares and concerns about:

## A Mother's Prayer for Week 26

Dear Father God,

I thank You for giving us spiritual insight through Your Word.

I pray that my baby will grow to have sharp spiritual vision. May he or she experience Your calling on his or her life at an early age. Open the eyes of my child's heart and enlighten his or her mind with Your Word. Fill my baby's life with the glorious riches that are the inheritance of Your people. Fill his or her life with love, joy, peace, patience, kindness, goodness, and temperance. As a parent, I stand for my child in prayer and claim the promises in the Bible for him or her.

And, Lord, I pray for my baby's eyes, that they will open and see this week or sometime very soon, according to what is right for his or her development. Please give my child perfect vision. If there is anything that threatens my baby's sight, I ask You to heal it right now and create a perfect retina, a perfect optic nerve, and perfect interpretation of the image displayed in his or her brain.

And, Lord, I pray that if I'm having twins, they will have a special relationship and become close friends right from the beginning. Give them a bond that cannot be broken.

In Jesus' name. Amen.

# Week 27

You will keep him in perfect peace,
Whose mind is stayed on You,
Because he trusts in You.

Isaiah 26:3 NKJV

As your pregnancy progresses, it may become more difficult to get a good night's rest. There are multiple reasons you may have trouble sleeping at some point in the nine months of your pregnancy. Here are 15 common sleep stealers:

1. Can't get comfortable
2. Exercise before bed keying you up
3. Frequent trips to the bathroom
4. Heartburn and indigestion
5. Hunger
6. Insomnia
7. Leg cramps
8. Medications
9. Nausea
10. Restless legs syndrome
11. Sharing a bed
12. Sleep apnea
13. Snoring and congestion
14. Vivid dreams
15. Worrying about your baby

I experienced 13 of the 15 listed here. The funniest one was the restless legs syndrome. One night, my husband woke me up and said I was kicking him. Of course, I didn't remember anything. The next night, I woke up with three big pillows in between us. I guess he was serious!

I love what Jesus said about being worn out: "Come to Me, all of you who are weary and burdened, and I will give you rest" (Matt. 11:28). Psalm 4:8 says, "I will both lie down and sleep in peace, for You alone, LORD, make me live in safety."

Do you feel weary and burdened? Any anxiety that we have, we can give to God. Any worries we have about our baby's sleep, we can just ask God to give us peace about them and He will.

After Micah was born, the first question I remember people asking was if my baby was sleeping through the night. Since he was my first baby, I never thought of praying for his sleep while I was pregnant, and it seemed that he practically never slept. He woke up almost every hour to nurse for the entire first year. It seemed that I had no choice but to keep him in my bed.

I didn't make the same mistake twice. With our daughter, Malia, I prayed and prayed for a good sleep pattern right from the beginning. And wouldn't you know it, God answered my prayer right away. The first week, she pretty much slept the whole time, which is normal, but by the second week, she gave me six to eight hours of sleep a night. It was wonderful! Once she started teething, well, that's another story.

Sleep, or lack of it, affects your ability to function, and it affects your baby's growth. This week, ask for God's grace and for restful sleep for you and your baby.

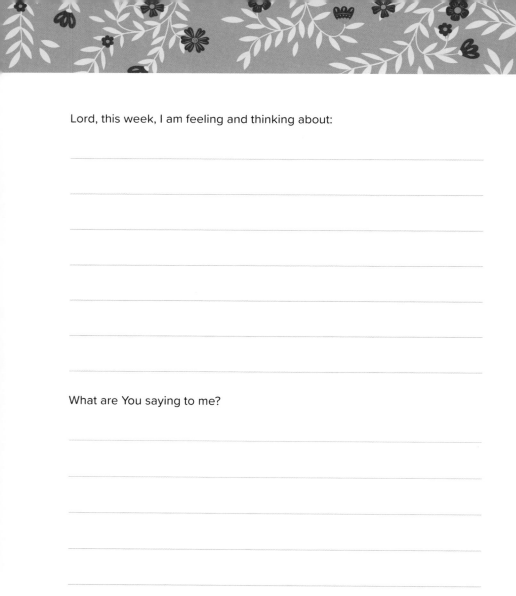

Lord, this week, I am feeling and thinking about:

What are You saying to me?

Read Psalm 23; Proverbs 3:5–8; Matthew 6:25–27; Philippians 4:6–7; 1 Peter 5:7–11.

Some of the things God has to say about worry and the antidote to it:

This week, I release to God my cares and concerns about:

## A Mother's Prayer for Week 27

Dear Lord,

You gave us sleep as a time for rest and renewal. You showed us by example when You created the world and took the seventh day to rest. Lord, please help me, tonight and from this time forward, to get a deep and rejuvenating sleep. If I wake up in the middle of the night, please help me to go right back to sleep.

Lord, please help my baby to develop good sleep patterns from the very beginning. I pray for safety while my baby sleeps. Protect him or her from SIDS or any other harm. Let your angels watch over him or her all through the night—and the daytime too.

Bless my baby, whether in his or her crib, by my side, or in the car seat or stroller. Anywhere he or she sleeps, make it relaxing and peaceful.

Lord, You promise us in Isaiah 26:3 that You'll keep our minds in perfect peace when we trust in You. Help me keep my focus and trust in You and cast out all fears. I choose peace of mind. I choose to trust in You, Lord Jesus, because I know You love me and my baby with an everlasting love. I receive Your peace right now.

Thank You, Jesus. Amen.

Third Trimester

# Weeks 28 to Birth

All the days ordained for me were written in your book before one of them came to be.

Psalm 139:16 NIV

# Week 28

> Don't worry about anything, but in everything, through prayer and petition with thanksgiving, let your requests be made known to God. And the peace of God, which surpasses every thought, will guard your hearts and minds in Christ Jesus.
>
> Philippians 4:6–7

The third trimester means your baby is almost here! Now it's time to create a birth plan to prepare for your labor and delivery. You may already know how you'd like the birth experience to go, but there are many choices and options to consider.

The best plan is to have a plan, so start jotting down ideas now and get your husband and health care provider involved too. Here are some things to consider:

- Where do I hope my baby's birth will take place? At a hospital, at a birthing center, or at home?
- Do I want to be able to move around during labor?
- Do I want to drink fluids during labor?
- Do I prefer an IV, or do I want a heparin or saline lock for any fluids and medications?
- What medication will I use, or do I prefer natural childbirth?
- What birthing positions would I like?
- Who will be allowed in the room with me?
- What will I wear?
- Do I want music played? Scriptures read?
- Do I want the room to be quiet? Would I like the lights dimmed?
- Am I comfortable with medical students or others in training being present?

- Do I want someone to take photos or videos of the birth?
- Will I breastfeed my baby soon after the birth?
- Is it okay if the hospital gives my baby formula?
- If it's a boy, will he be circumcised?

By creating a birth plan, you'll have peace of mind knowing that your preferences are clearly spelled out. Yes, something unexpected may come up, and if it helps, you can even create what-ifs in your birth plan. You can make changes as you work through your ideas, and when you're finished, print out copies for your practitioner, nurse, doula, and husband, and one to keep for your baby book.

But before the birth, let's take a look at the last trimester. During this time, a baby swallows up to a liter a day of amniotic fluid, and scientists believe this may serve as a "flavor bridge" to consuming his or her mother's milk, which is also influenced by flavors from the food the mother eats. God set it up so your baby will automatically like the taste of your breast milk. Isn't that amazing?

Lord, this week, I am feeling and thinking about:

What are You saying to me?

This week, I'm grateful to God for:

This week, I release to God my cares and concerns about:

## A Mother's Prayer for Week 28

Dear Lord Jesus,

Thank You for helping me make it this far in my pregnancy, and for the way You will help me through these final months. Help me increase my prayer time and hear Your Holy Spirit as You speak to me. Help me recognize Your voice and understand what You say. Continue to teach me to be open to You and to trust in You.

And, Lord, protect me from complications in pregnancy. Safeguard my health and my baby's health. Protect me from unnecessary scares and fear. Lord, Your Word says perfect love casts out fear (1 John 4:18). I accept Your love and the peace of the Holy Spirit. I put my life in Your hands, and I will not fear.

I pray for my baby's continued growth during this final trimester. Lead and guide me as I prepare my birth plan.

I praise Your holy name, Jesus. Amen.

# Week 29

My sheep hear my voice, and I know them, and they follow me. I give them eternal life, and they will never perish, and no one will snatch them out of my hand.

John 10:27–28 ESV

Newborn babies recognize their mother's voice. Let's think about that. How can a baby recognize his or her mother's voice five seconds after birth? The logical line of thought is that the baby must have been able to hear his or her mother speaking before birth. True enough, but the science community did not have hard evidence that this was so until an exciting, groundbreaking research project took place among 60 pregnant women.

Here's what happened: The mothers-to-be read a two-minute poem into a recorder. Half of the unborn babies heard the voices of their mothers reading the poem; the other half heard the same poem read by a woman other than their mothers. The question was, would the babies react differently to the sound of their own mother's voice when the same words were played?

When the recording of the mother's voice was held next to her abdomen, her baby's heart rate increased throughout the entire recording and remained high for the next two minutes as well. But when another woman's voice was played at the same volume, the baby's heart rate decreased and remained lower throughout and after the recording. In both groups, the changes to the babies' heart rates began about 20 seconds into the recording, which shows they were reacting to the recording.

According to lead researcher Barbara Kisilevsky, PhD, of Queen's University in Ontario, Canada, "They get excited when they hear their mother's voice; it is something that they recognize and are aroused by. What this study shows is that the babies had to recognize and distinguish between the two voices in order to respond differently."[1]

In a different research project, Anthony DeCasper, PhD, psychologist at the University of North Carolina, discovered that babies react differently to different stories, even when read by the same mother.[2] That tells me the babies recognize their own mother's voice, and they distinguish between messages.

I don't know about you, but I think this is a lot of exciting proof—and a big dose of inspiration to pray aloud for our babies and to read the Bible aloud. If you're wondering where to start in reading the Bible, I suggest reading the book of Mark in the New Testament, because it's only 16 chapters and it tells the story of Jesus. Then I recommend reading some of the Psalms. Many are beautiful poems and songs inspired by God, and they are a great place to go when you are hurting or scared.

Babies recognizing and responding to their own mother's voice reminds me of when Jesus said His people know His voice and follow Him (John 10:27). That's what I want for my children also—to recognize the voice of Jesus and follow Him.

Lord, this week, I am feeling and thinking about:

_____

_____

_____

_____

_____

_____

What are You saying to me?

_____

_____

_____

_____

_____

_____

_____

Write out a special message to your baby and then read it aloud. When your child is older, you can look back and read it again together. This is about creating a beautiful moment for you to share together in the future.

This week, I release to God my cares and concerns about:

_____

_____

_____

_____

_____

_____

_____

_____

_____

_____

_____

_____

_____

_____

## A Mother's Prayer for Week 29

Dear Lord,

I pray for my baby's hearing that is developing now. Give him or her perfect hearing, with the ears and inner parts of the ear working properly. And, Lord, I also pray that my child will hear and recognize Your voice. Give him or her spiritual ears to hear what You are saying to my child's generation, and to him or her specifically. I pray that my child will love Your voice and be sensitive to it.

Lord, You say in the Gospel of John that Your people hear You and follow You, and that You give them eternal life. I pray now for my child's salvation, that You would give my child a wonderful experience in knowing You are his or her personal Lord and Savior and that You have prepared eternal life for him or her.

Lord, I also pray that my words express love and are positive, encouraging, life-giving, and Bible-based. I pray that my baby hears only good things coming out of my mouth, and I pray that I will think about what I am going to say before I say it. Help me teach by my words and actions.

Show my child the path in which You want him or her to go, and help my child to spread the Good News of Jesus Christ wherever he or she goes.

Thank You for hearing my prayer.

In Jesus' name. Amen.

# Week 30

I have learned to be content in whatever circumstances I am.

Philippians 4:11

This week, and in the last trimester, you may start to experience fatigue again, like you did in the first trimester. Between carrying the weight of your baby and not sleeping well, it's to be expected. Do let your health care provider know, though, so they can rule out any other possibilities.

This is a good time to focus on your health, for you and the baby. Some women feel like they're being self-centered when they take time out for themselves to exercise, but that's not true. Your baby also benefits when you exercise. What's more, you need to take care of yourself if you're going to be able to take good care of your child. Even now, I try not to feel bad about doing something good for myself, because I know it helps me be a more patient mother.

Swimming is an awesome way for pregnant women to exercise. With the water's buoyancy, you become virtually weightless, reducing stress on your joints. Swimming a few laps works all major muscle groups, your heart, and your lungs. You can enjoy whatever strokes you feel comfortable with—breaststroke, sidestroke, front crawl, or backstroke—as long as you don't strain yourself.

Water jogging or walking is also an awesome workout for your legs and cardiovascular system. It's a good idea to stay about waist deep.

Another advantage of water exercise is that the water helps prevent you from becoming overheated.

However you decide to exercise, anytime that you feel yourself getting too hot, make sure to stop, drink some water, and rest. Do not let your heart rate exceed 120 beats per minute. Stop immediately and call your doctor if you start having contractions, and always follow the exercise directions given to you by your doctor or health care provider.

How hard can you work out during pregnancy? On a scale of 1 to 10, with 1 being "no challenge" and 10 being "extremely difficult," go for a level of 4 to 5 right now, because you're in your third trimester and don't want to overdo it. The key here is just to get up and move every day.

Another way you can help your fatigue—and your baby's skeletal structure to grow strong—is by getting enough protein, calcium, and iron.

Your baby relies on you for all his or her iron, which is stored up to last for the first six months of life. If you lack iron, your baby will be served first, and then you may suffer from fatigue, headaches, and difficulty concentrating. Fortunately, your body absorbs calcium better now than before you were pregnant—thank God for that—especially in this last half of pregnancy, when your baby needs the most calcium and is growing rapidly.

It's easier to have patience when you're taking care of your body and feeling good. It's hard to wait so long for your baby to come, especially if you're not feeling well, but you can rely on the Lord to give you patience. Think of Romans 5:3–4: "Suffering produces endurance, and endurance produces character, and character produces hope" (ESV).

When you feel like you're suffering with various discomforts due to pregnancy, realize that you are building endurance and character, and then take comfort in the hope that it will all be worth it when you hold your baby in your arms.

But remember, it takes time and practice to build patience—so don't be impatient! Just keep trusting in the Lord.

Lord, this week, I am feeling and thinking about:

_____

_____

_____

_____

_____

_____

What are You saying to me?

_____

_____

_____

_____

_____

_____

I can help teach my child to build patience by:

This week, I release to God my cares and concerns about:

## A Mother's Prayer for Week 30

Dear Lord,

I praise You for the hard times that stretch my endurance, because I know they're producing good character and working out patience in me. Help me apply Hebrews 12:1: "Let us run with patience the race that is set before us" (KJV). I know that applies spiritually, but right now, it also applies to waiting out the time before my baby comes.

I pray that You will help me manifest patience in our home, so that my child will grow up with a good role model. Give my baby a patient spirit, and may he or she be slow to anger and quick to praise.

Lord, please continue to help my baby grow strong in every way. And help me take the time to be healthy.

In Jesus' name. Amen.

# Week 31

We have peace with God through our Lord Jesus Christ.

Romans 5:1

By this time, all your baby's major organs are developed, but the lungs still need to mature in order for your baby to breathe on his or her own. From here until the birth, your baby will gain weight and strengthen his or her immune system in preparation for life on the outside. Your baby's immune system is still not fully mature at birth, but God provided a way for you to help. The antibodies made by your own body's immune system are passed on to your baby when you breastfeed, protecting against many different diseases and illnesses. It is also a wonderful bonding experience! There are valid reasons why some women cannot or choose not to breastfeed their babies, and millions of babies who were fed formula are strong, healthy, and doing very well. So please know that I support the personal decision of all mothers. But my own personal belief is that, ideally, God created mothers to nurse their babies, so I encourage you to consider this option.

In addition to praying for your baby's health and immune system, pray that your baby is peaceful and has a calm spirit. We live in a world filled with stress and bad news. Many people live in fear of what could happen. Yes, bad things happen in the world, which seems to be getting worse each day, but we can stand securely on the promises of God and be confident in Jesus as our Protector.

First John 4:4 says, "You are from God, little children . . . because the One who is in you is greater than the one who is in the world."

Jesus is called the Prince of Peace (see Isa. 9:6). Let's pray for our little ones to be calm, peaceful babies and to grow up with an inner peace that comes from above.

Jesus said, "My peace I give to you. I do not give to you as the world gives. Your heart must not be troubled or fearful" (John 14:27). I'd like to share with you an interesting insight on experiencing peace through silence from Elmer L. Towns, dean emeritus at Liberty University and a Gold Medallion award-winning author. In his book *How to Pray When You Don't Know What to Say*, Towns writes:

> Do you know that there is power in silence? The power of silence comes not from the absence of words but from the presence of God. When we are silent before God, the Lord can heal us, or build us up, or make us what He intended for us to be: "My soul, wait silently for God alone, for my expectation is from Him" (Ps. 62:5).[1]

We don't have to bang on the door or yell to get God's attention. Too often we think of silence as the absence of noise or just nothing in the room. But silence is something. Silence has its own existence. Just as God exists without being a physical presence, so silence exists for us. When we enter the stillness of our personal sanctuary, we'll find that God is there. He is waiting for us in our silence.[2]

It's usually the mom who sets the mood for the household. When we slow down long enough to enjoy the peace of God, we can share it with others.

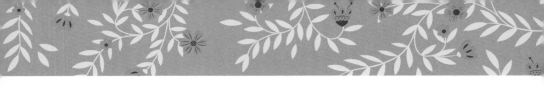

Lord, this week, I am feeling and thinking about:

_____

_____

_____

_____

_____

_____

_____

What are You saying to me?

_____

_____

_____

_____

_____

_____

_____

If I need to work on something in my heart, I will ask the Lord to bring it to my attention. I can create peace and harmony in our home by taking these concrete actions and creating this kind of atmosphere:

This week, I release to God my cares and concerns about:

## A Mother's Prayer for Week 31

Dear Lord Jesus,

Thank You for the privilege of knowing You. Thank You for the peace You give. Lord, I come to You, not frantic or worrying, but with a calm spirit, knowing You are here with me.

I pray that my baby will be born into a peaceful, calm atmosphere and have a peaceful, calm spirit. Help my child to grow up knowing You and having Your peace in his or her heart, no matter what situations my child encounters.

Lord, help me create a secure, calm, peaceful atmosphere in our home—one where love can thrive.

And, dear Lord, I pray that my baby will develop a strong immune system. Protect my child from disease and illness. Help me feed my baby the best way I can. Whether it's by breastfeeding or by bottle, help my baby to get the nourishment he or she needs on a daily basis.

I praise You and thank You.

In Jesus' name. Amen.

# Week 32

Rejoice in the Lord always. I will say it again: Rejoice! Let your graciousness be known to everyone. The Lord is near. Don't worry about anything, but in everything, through prayer and petition with thanksgiving, let your requests be made known to God. And the peace of God, which surpasses every thought, will guard your hearts and minds in Christ Jesus.

Philippians 4:4–7

Your baby's skin is looking more beautiful this week. The allover baby hair is disappearing, and the skin is enviably smooth.

This is a good time to pray that your baby won't develop any of the common newborn baby skin disorders, such as cradle cap or infant acne, even though they aren't serious. God cares for every small detail of our lives, not just the major issues. He knows our thoughts, what we want and need, and everything we go through. Some people fear that God is too busy for "little issues" like temporary rashes, but that's not so. That type of thinking is actually an insult to God, because it puts a limit on His ability to show us compassion and give us good gifts.

God doesn't get "too busy." God is all-powerful and ever-present. He can handle a billion prayer requests at once as easily as He can handle one. God is GOD. He does not experience the limitations of humans, and this means we must not limit our faith in Him or be afraid that our request is too small to "bother" Him with.

If it concerns you, it concerns God, because He loves you.

Think about it this way: If your son or daughter came to you with a burning, itchy rash, would you say, "I'm too busy to think about your pain and suffering"? Or would you say, "That's no big deal; don't bother me with it"? No, of course not. You would stop to look at the rash, pray over it, and do what you could to make it better. The Scriptures say that if you—being a mere human and a sinner—know how to treat your child right and give that child what he or she needs, don't you think your great and loving God knows how to do the same? Of course! God, who is perfect and is not only loving but also Love, will do even better. So never hesitate to ask the Lord for what you and your baby need. Remember, Philippians 4:6 says, "Don't worry about anything, but in everything, through prayer and petition with thanksgiving, let your requests be made known to God."

## A Prayer for Joy

In addition to your baby's skin, pray for your baby to have joy. We don't live in a perfect world; we expect to go through troubles in this life. God clearly says that in this world we will have tribulation, but that doesn't mean we have to let our joy slip away.

Pray that your child will grow up having a joyful spirit. I love what Nehemiah 8:10 says: "The joy of the LORD is your strength" (NIV).

Isn't that fantastic? Our source of strength can be joy! I have to tell you I prayed diligently for our son to have a spirit of joy, and now everywhere we go, people comment on what a joyful, happy spirit he has. Because their comments are exactly in line with what I prayed for, I take it as an answer to prayer. So be encouraged to pray the same for your baby.

Lord, this week, I am feeling and thinking about:

_____

_____

_____

_____

_____

_____

_____

What are You saying to me?

_____

_____

_____

_____

_____

_____

_____

I would like my child to find true joy in his or her early life because:

_____

_____

_____

_____

_____

_____

I know God finds joy in me and my baby because:

_____

_____

_____

_____

_____

_____

This week, I release to God my cares and concerns about:

## A Mother's Prayer for Week 32

Dear Lord,

I pray for my baby's skin. Help it to grow soft and beautiful, the way a baby's skin is supposed to be. And because You said to ask for what we want, I'm asking You to protect my baby from getting any bad skin disorders. Protect him or her from getting infant acne, cradle cap, jaundice, and diaper rashes. Lord, I know those are common skin conditions, but based on Your Word that tells us You care for each and every detail of our lives, I pray that You will protect my baby from those. Give me wisdom and knowledge to do the right things to protect his or her skin. Help me know which foods and products to avoid so that I can help my child. Help me be a good parent and give my child all the care he or she needs.

But, Lord, even more importantly, I pray that You will fill my child's heart and life with joy. Give my child the joy of the Lord and help him or her to find inner strength as a result of that joy. In all situations, let the joy of the Lord be in my child's heart. And, Lord, help me to be a role model of joy in my home. Help me bring a spirit of joy into our house.

I love You, Lord, because You are good and because You are all-powerful and ever-present. Thank You for caring about every detail of my life. I know You are never too busy to hear my prayers, because You are GOD, and You can do all things. You delight in giving good gifts to Your children. You care for us, and I receive that.

In Jesus' name. Amen.

# Week 33

I will praise You as long as I live;
at Your name, I will lift up my hands. . . .
When I think of You as I lie on my bed,
I meditate on You during the night watches
because You are my helper;
I will rejoice in the shadow of Your wings.
I follow close to You;
Your right hand holds on to me.

Psalm 63:4, 6–8

The headline this week for your baby is GROWTH. Not only is he or she steadily gaining weight, but your baby is also continuing to put on the fat that's necessary to cope with the climate on the outside. The brain is rapidly growing and maturing as well.

Most babies will gain five to nine ounces every week from week 33 until birth.

During this period of tremendous physical growth, it's a good time to focus on growing in faith too. While I was writing this book, I received this beautiful letter from Barb Rickford of Colorado:

> When I still wasn't pregnant at the age of forty, I thought it wasn't going to happen, that it wasn't in God's will. But then while I was in the process of letting go, I discovered I was pregnant at age 41. Since my journey to become a mom was long and difficult, I've learned the importance and the power of prayer—not only during pregnancy but also before conception and following right through the birth.
>
> Like Hannah, I prayed for my child, and the Lord granted me what I asked of Him, in His perfect time. So whenever I came across a Bible verse I felt pertained to my child, I prayed it and then wrote the date

in my Bible. God promises that His Word, spoken in faith, will not return void, and will accomplish His purpose (see Isa. 55:11). These are a few of the Scriptures and prayers that guided me in speaking blessing into my child's life—and they still guide me to this day:

*Passion:* Lord, please instill in my child a soul with a heart for You; a heart that clings passionately to You (Ps. 63:8); and the things that are good, true, noble, lovely, excellent, and praiseworthy (see Phil. 4:8).

*Purpose:* Lord, I pray that my child's life will serve Your purpose in his own generation (see Acts 13:36; Esther 4:14).

*Faith:* Lord, I pray that faith will find root and grow in my child's heart and that by faith my child may gain what has been promised to him (see Luke 17:5–6; Heb. 11:1–40). Reveal Yourself to my child at an early age (see 1 Sam. 3:7).

*Favor:* Lord, I pray that my child will grow in stature and favor with You and with men (see 1 Sam. 2:26).

*Courage:* Lord, may my child always "be strong and courageous" in his character and actions (see Deut. 31:6).

*Contentment:* Lord, teach my child "the secret of being content" in any and every situation as You give him strength (see Phil. 4:12–13).

Barb ended her letter by explaining that she believes God's gift of pregnancy wasn't because she deserved this incredible blessing, but that it was God's way of showing His love and His perfect timing. She said, "I've never been filled with such awe and wonder; it was the most euphoric, fulfilling day of my life. Prayer is powerful!"

Lord, this week, I am feeling and thinking about:

_____

_____

_____

_____

_____

_____

What are You saying to me?

_____

_____

_____

_____

_____

_____

_____

Lord, where do I need to grow in my faith this week? Where do I need to trust You? I will show that my passion and purpose are in You by:

This week, I release to God my cares and concerns about:

## A Mother's Prayer for Week 33

Dear Lord,

I pray that my baby will find his or her passion and purpose in life. Lead and guide my child right from the start, and reveal Your will to him or her at an early age. Make Your will clear and help my child never to veer off course from the plan You have for his or her life.

Help my child obey Your Word and grow in favor with You and with people, so that he or she might prosper and be blessed.

Give my child courage in the face of difficulty. Be his or her strength and strong tower, as it says in Proverbs 18:10. I pray that my child keeps focused on You and is fearless, because You are with him or her.

Grant my child contentment, so that he or she has a happy heart.

And, Lord, I thank You so much for the blessing of being pregnant with this child. Your Word says every good and perfect gift comes from above. I acknowledge You as the giver of life. I am looking forward to meeting this baby You have given me. I will praise You for as long as I live.

In Jesus' name. Amen.

Give thanks to Yahweh, call on His name;
proclaim His deeds among the peoples.

Psalm 105:1

Being grateful is the way we should live as followers of Christ. It's being happy over what you've been given, rather than being discontent about what you don't have. I like the idea of keeping a Happiness Journal in which you write down something that made you happy that day. For example, your happy moment might be the sighting of a hummingbird, or it could be that you finally got caught up on the laundry. Whatever it is, writing it down is a tangible way of living a life of gratitude and remembering the gifts you've been given.

I am so grateful for my six siblings. Please don't feel bad if your own situation is different. Even if you don't have blood brothers or sisters, you have the Body of Christ. God can fill the void by giving you Christian friends. He has provided a way for us to be a part of His family and to be able to give and receive the support we need. Ephesians 2:19 says that we are "members of God's household." Now that's a wonderful household to be a part of!

My mother, a woman I love and admire for the way that she tapped into God's strength to raise her four boys and three girls, wrote me about her own prayer habits during pregnancy:

*I remember praying a lot during each of my pregnancies, but I can't remember all the specifics in regards to what I prayed for each child. (I wish I'd kept a journal.) But I do remember praying for each of you: "Lord, please bless my baby with wisdom and a strong, sound mind. Let him or her be healthy and whole (with 10 fingers and 10 toes, and no abnormalities). Help him or her to grow close to You and trust in You as Savior. Help my baby to become a righteous man or woman who wants to serve You and serve others ahead of himself or herself."*

*For some of you, I prayed for your future spouse while you were still in the womb, asking the Lord to bring the special person He had chosen for you into your life at precisely the right time.*

*For others I prayed, "Heavenly Father, please use my child to spread the gospel around the world to every nation. Help my child to always seek first Your kingdom and Your righteousness. Help him or her to be a witness for You, and give my child a desire to do Your will."*

*God has answered all these petitions, and many more; He has blessed me and our family far more than I ever envisioned.*

Lord, this week, I am feeling and thinking about:

_____

_____

_____

_____

_____

_____

What are You saying to me?

_____

_____

_____

_____

_____

_____

_____

What God wants me to record in my Happiness Journal today:

_____

_____

_____

_____

_____

What makes me happy about carrying my child:

_____

_____

_____

_____

_____

_____

I am blessed to be a part of God's family. People I am close to:

This week, I release to God my cares and concerns about:

## A Mother's Prayer for Week 34

Dear Lord,

Please bless my baby with wisdom and a strong, sound mind. Let him or her be healthy and whole (with 10 fingers and 10 toes, and no abnormalities). Help him or her to grow close to You and trust in You as Savior. Help my child to become a righteous man or woman who wants to serve You and serve others ahead of himself or herself.

I pray for my child's future spouse. I ask You to bring the special person You have chosen for my child into his or her life at precisely the right time.

Heavenly Father, please use my child to spread the gospel around the world to every nation. Help my child to always seek first Your kingdom and Your righteousness. Help him or her to be a witness for You, and give my child a desire to do Your will.

I ask you to bless my family far more than I could ever envision!

In Jesus' name. Amen.

# Week 35

You're probably thinking a lot about your baby's arrival; hopefully, you're not embarking on other big projects at the same time!

This week, your baby weighs about five pounds or more, but he or she still needs to add fat in order to keep warm enough after birth. Babies born at thirty-five weeks are usually put in an incubator for added warmth while they grow. Nevertheless, it's getting snug in your womb, so he or she doesn't have as much room for doing gymnastics as before. You might notice that your baby is more active when you're resting and quieter when you're moving around. This is because you are virtually rocking him or her to sleep with your movements.

Soon, you'll be rocking him or her in your arms, so it makes sense to prepare for the delivery at this time.

## Get Ready!

This is a good time to make a list so that you won't forget something essential, like your phone to take pictures and videos with, when that big day finally comes. I also recommend packing your bag to take to the hospital or birthing center now, just in case your baby decides to surprise you with an early debut! I like to tell moms-to-be, "Expect the unexpected." At the end of this book, we've included a suggested list of what to take to the hospital, but here are just a few items to start with:

- Copies of your birth plan
- Nursing bras and pads

- Nighttime sanitary napkins
- Clothes to wear when visitors come to take pictures
- Personal toiletries, including lip moisturizer
- Cell phone with camera
- Bible
- Uplifting music on your playlist
- Hair tie
- Stretchy, comfortable clothes to wear home, such as sweatpants and a T-shirt
- Flip-flops or easy slide-in shoes
- Clothes for your baby to wear home
- Baby blankets
- Baby car seat for travel home (required)

A few comments about clothes to bring: The hospital will provide a gown, but many hospitals will allow you to wear your own clothes if you prefer. If you live in a cold climate, you might also want warm socks. For your going-home outfit, bring something you fit into when you were about six months pregnant, because it takes a little time for your body to shrink back to its original shape and size. And leave your jewelry at home.

Having your bag packed will be one less last-minute thing you have to do. Other suggestions for getting ready are to have your house in order—my husband really took that one to heart!—and to have the laundry done if possible. I know some mothers suggest getting a good haircut before the birth, because it will be a while before you can make it into the salon afterward.

Lord, this week, I am feeling and thinking about:

_____

_____

_____

_____

_____

_____

What are You saying to me?

_____

_____

_____

_____

_____

_____

My list of things to do before my baby arrives:

This week, I release to God my cares and concerns about:

## A Mother's Prayer for Week 35

Dear Lord Jesus,

I thank You for my baby and that I've made it this far in my pregnancy.

Lord, I pray that Your Holy Spirit would come right now into the place where I am. Let me receive Your holy presence right now. Jesus, I pray that You will bless me with joy and gladness as I prepare for my baby's birth. Help me remember what I've learned in my birth classes and what I've read. Help me remember the Scriptures that apply to me. Make Your Word a living testament to me.

Bless my husband too, and help him to be the strong support that I need. Bless my other children with love and gladness.

Help me get through these last weeks with a minimal amount of discomfort. Help me sleep through the night in peace. Strengthen me in preparation for the wonderful event of my baby's birth. Give me a quick and manageable delivery, and help this baby to be healthy and perfect in every way.

In Jesus' wonderful name I pray. Amen.

# Week 36

Shout triumphantly to the LORD, all the earth.
Serve the LORD with gladness;
come before Him with joyful songs.
Acknowledge that Yahweh is God.
He made us, and we are His—
His people, the sheep of His pasture.
Enter His gates with thanksgiving
and His courts with praise.
Give thanks to Him and praise His name.
For Yahweh is good, and His love is eternal;
His faithfulness endures through all generations.

Psalm 100

Your baby is getting ready to meet you! By the end of the week, your baby will be considered full term and capable of surviving on his or her own. Perhaps the most important event for your baby this week is that he or she stops floating freely and gets into the birth position. Once in position, a baby usually limits his or her movements to rolling from side to side.

If you're carrying twins, your babies' birthday could be this week. The National Organization of Mothers of Twins Clubs says the average twin birth occurs between 36 and 37 weeks, and the babies weigh an average of five pounds each.

At this point, a mom-to-be has one main thing on her mind, which is—you guessed it—*My baby is almost here!* By now, you've read technical and medical information about everything that's happening with your body, and even about all the things that could possibly go wrong. There's a wealth of information to discover, but I ask you this: When do you read that you can experience God's presence in the delivery room? When do you hear about bringing your baby into a room filled with the prayers and praises of Jesus? And what about having the Word of God spoken to you as encouragement while you're in labor? I can't help but believe this is the way it should be!

Whether your baby comes at home, in a birthing center, in a hospital, or on the operating table via C-section, the Lord's sweet presence can be right there with you in a real way.

We read in God's Word over and over again that the Lord dwells in the praises of His people. Psalm 22:3 says that the Lord inhabits praise. So when we pray and praise Him, His presence comes to us. That's a promise and a spiritual law.

Has it occurred to you that God might come into your delivery room and surround you with His peace and love and make your delivery the most wonderful spiritual experience you've ever had? This week, pray that our loving Lord and Savior, Jesus Christ, will be right with you, lifting you up into His love during your labor, and that your baby will be born into a room that is filled with His peace and joy.

Lord, this week, I am feeling and thinking about:

_____

_____

_____

_____

_____

_____

What are You saying to me?

_____

_____

_____

_____

_____

_____

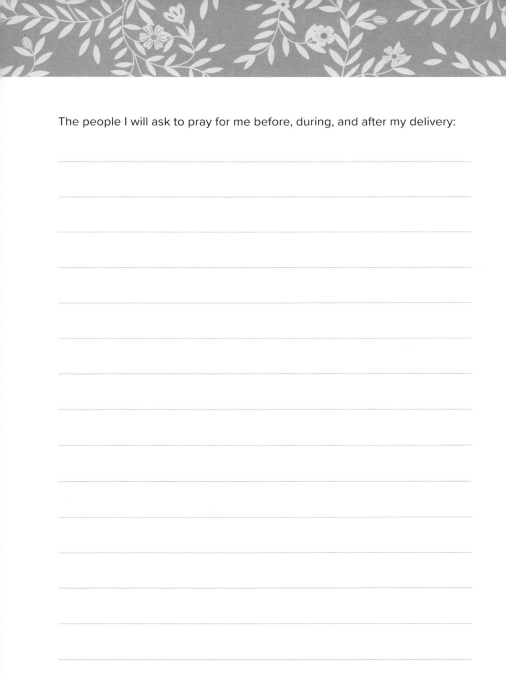

The people I will ask to pray for me before, during, and after my delivery:

This week, I release to God my cares and concerns about:

## A Mother's Prayer for Week 36

Dear Lord Jesus,

Thank You for the privilege of knowing You as my personal Savior and Friend. I praise You because You are a great and wonderful God, full of love and care and understanding.

Lord, I pray that You will give me the most wonderful birth experience I could imagine. Be close to me from the time I go into labor and throughout. Let me feel You lift me up into Your love during each contraction. Let me know You are with me, helping and guiding my baby to be born. Give me strength and endurance.

And, Jesus, I pray Your holy presence will fill the room as my baby comes into this world. Let there be an atmosphere of joy and gladness, of peace and praise.

Give me an awesome birth experience, one I will treasure forever.

In Jesus' name. Amen.

# Week 37

Cast all your anxiety on him because he cares for you.

1 Peter 5:7 NIV

No matter what news you may get about your baby, God is there with you. Jesus said, "I will never abandon you or leave you" (Heb. 13:5 GW). God is good. At first, the news may be devastating to you, but the Lord always has a plan.

Week 37 was a test of faith for me during my second pregnancy. I found out my baby was breech, and I was facing a procedure that could cause the water bag to break. If that occurred, they'd have to perform an emergency C-section.

Dan and I tried all the options to get the baby to turn, even the ones that seemed a bit weird. All week I prayed, but the baby didn't turn. I sent emails asking for prayer, and our pastor prayed with us. I felt the baby moving around, but I wasn't sure.

The day of my doctor's appointment to turn the baby manually arrived. We waited while they set up to do an emergency C-section, just in case it was needed. I thought, *What if I have my baby today!* I wasn't ready for that yet.

The resident doctor placed the scanner on my tummy, and just a couple of seconds later, I took a deep breath and the doctor announced, "Your baby's head is down!"

I exclaimed, "Really? Thank You, God!" We were all so excited! God was working on our behalf. We thanked Him and gave Him all the glory.

Interestingly, when our pastor had prayed for me at home, he had a strong feeling that the baby would turn, and he was right. I might have felt it that morning in bed—a gentle, swishy feeling like a fish swimming along my belly. I kept thinking, *Wow, God answered those prayers too!* With bolstered faith and praises in our hearts, we went home and waited for our daughter to come—when she was ready.

You may be feeling Braxton Hicks contractions, or false labor, strongly this week. If so, don't be alarmed as the contractions work to help prepare your body for birth.

Here are some tips to distinguish pre-labor contractions from the real thing:

- True contractions grow stronger and closer together, and they last longer.
- True contractions don't go away if you lie down or relax in a warm tub.
- Braxton Hicks tend to be felt only in front and not all over.
- Walking has no effect on Braxton Hicks, whereas it makes true contractions stronger.
- The cervix doesn't change with Braxton Hicks, whereas it opens and thins with true labor.

If you have contractions, follow the instructions you've been given by your doctor. Each woman is unique, and your doctor knows your individual pregnancy history and will have instructions for when to call.

Lord, this week, I am feeling and thinking about:

_____

_____

_____

_____

_____

_____

What are You saying to me?

_____

_____

_____

_____

_____

_____

Matthew 11:29–30 says, "All of you, take up My yoke and learn from Me, because I am gentle and humble in heart, and you will find rest for yourselves. For My yoke is easy and My burden is light." This is what that passage means to me:

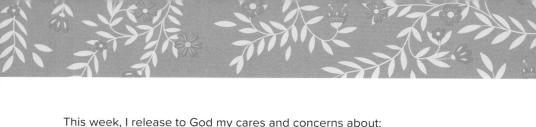

This week, I release to God my cares and concerns about:

## A Mother's Prayer for Week 37

Dear Lord,

You are almighty and know everything that is going on with my body and my baby. You know the exact minute that my baby is coming.

Lord, this has been a season of learning to trust in You more. Your ways are higher than our ways, and Your thoughts are higher than ours. I place myself and my child in Your hands and trust in You alone. I know I can do all things You require of me, with Your help.

You are here with me now, every minute of the day and night. I know You will take care of my baby. Lord, I receive Your peace and I place my trust in You.

In Jesus' almighty name. Amen.

# Week 38

> She will give birth to a son, and you are to give him the name Jesus, because he will save his people from their sins.
>
> Matthew 1:21 NIV

Your baby could come any time now, or he or she could take a few more weeks to grow bigger and have his or her lungs develop just a bit more. God knows the exact minute your baby will be born, so try to be patient, double-check your list to make sure everything is ready, and then trust in Him.

This week, I want to share a story about a young woman who was engaged to be married and then discovered she was pregnant. This came as a complete surprise. She knew she had to tell her fiancé, and although he truly loved her, he became upset at this news and said he was breaking off the engagement. You see, she and her fiancé had not slept together; they had agreed to wait until they got married.

Now the young woman had to do something, because in her culture being an unmarried mother was not acceptable. In fact, a woman could even receive the death penalty for becoming pregnant outside of marriage. But here's something surprising. This woman went straight to visit her cousin, who happened to be married to the highest religious leader in the country—the very one who could issue the order to have her put to death.

She wasn't completely sure how her cousin would react, because her cousin had been wanting to get pregnant herself for many years and was now past menopause. But she hoped that her cousin Elizabeth would take her in and guard her life. At the very moment she arrived, Elizabeth— who had received a miracle from God and was now six months pregnant herself—exclaimed in a loud voice, "You are the most blessed of women, and your child will be blessed!"

The Holy Spirit had come upon Elizabeth, who spoke a word of prophecy. She continued, "How could this happen to me, that the mother of my Lord should come to me? For you see, when the sound of your greeting reached my ears, the baby leaped for joy inside me!" (Luke 1:43–44).

And you know the rest of this story. The young woman named Mary ended up staying with Elizabeth and her husband, Zechariah, the high priest, for three months, and then she returned safely to her home. In the meantime, the angel of the Lord showed up and informed Mary's fiancé that she had not been unfaithful but that she'd been chosen by God to be the mother of Jesus, the long-awaited Savior. Joseph must have been stunned, but what an honor to be the stepfather to Jesus! He and Mary went through with their plans and had the wedding.

But there was no honeymoon—not until after Jesus was born. So the prophecy was fulfilled that the Savior would be born of a virgin.

It's remarkable and beautiful that God would design a plan to rescue us from our own sinful doom through a virgin birth. On top of that, Mary's cousin Elizabeth also conceived when it was humanly impossible. She gave birth to John, commonly called John the Baptist, because he baptized Jesus in water at the start of Jesus' ministry.

This story—the most miraculous of all pregnancy and birth stories—is wonderful to consider as you prepare to give birth. This week, pray a prayer of thanksgiving to God for His wonderful Son.

Lord, this week, I am feeling and thinking about:

_____

_____

_____

_____

_____

_____

What are You saying to me?

_____

_____

_____

_____

_____

_____

What I love most about the story of Jesus' birth:

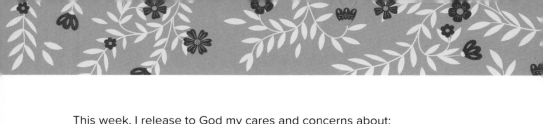

This week, I release to God my cares and concerns about:

## A Mother's Prayer for Week 38

Dear Lord God,

I thank You from the bottom of my heart for giving us Your Son, Jesus. It's such an amazing story, what You did for us. I pray You will give me courage and faith like Mary had.

And, Lord, only You know the exact minute my baby will be born. Please help me to be patient and get through this time of waiting. I am so anxious to see and hold my baby that I can barely wait another day. Please be close to me and surround me with Your love and presence at the birth. Help the labor go smoothly and the birth to go just right.

Thank You, Lord, for all You have done to provide us with a way to communicate with You. Thank You for salvation and for Your great love. Thank You for my baby.

In Jesus' name. Amen.

# Week 39

One week to go! If you're like me, you are so ready for your baby to be born. Some babies will arrive early. That's what happened with our second baby. (As you may recall from week 37, God miraculously turned her from being in the breech position to head-down after we prayed two weeks before her birth.)

Here's the rest of the story: Micah, now two and a half years old, and I were in the kitchen making breakfast, and I was still having contractions that began the night before. During every contraction I squatted down and did my deep-breathing exercises.

Dan arrived home from work that afternoon, took one look at me, and knew that today was the day. We prayed together, asking for a quick, safe, easy birth.

We drove to the doctor's office, and she gave us good news. Praise God, the baby was on the way! My contractions were now 10 minutes apart, and my doctor said to go home, get my bag, and then head for the hospital.

During the car ride the contractions increased and were more intense. We arrived at the hospital and settled into our room in "The Starting Place," a triage area.

The contractions progressed, and my baby was sitting low, fully engaged. At 6:40 p.m., I was in the cafeteria with Dan, our doula, Janet, and Micah, and I felt something weird. I thought my water bag broke, because all of a sudden, my contractions progressed quickly to about two minutes apart.

I said, "We need to go upstairs, NOW! This baby's coming."

Upstairs, I settled in to the "real" labor and delivery. The baby's heartbeat was doing great, and there were absolutely no signs of distress. Hallelujah!

Within what seemed like minutes of our arriving upstairs, the water bag broke again, and I said, "I feel like I want to push."

Our friends Claire and Pete showed up just in time to take care of Micah and relieve my doula of that duty. Janet traded places with Dan, who'd been doing a great job of coaching me up to that point.

I started pushing, and within 10 minutes our little girl was here. Praise God!

The Lord was with me through the entire time, and He answered my prayers for a smooth, fast delivery.

What an indescribable experience it was to meet my daughter and cuddle her close to me. My heart was filled with love. God truly had grace on me that day, and that's why Malia's middle name is Grace. Dan cried with joy when he saw his baby daughter. "It's a girl, my little girl," he said. I think we all cried then, overcome with happiness and gratitude to the Lord. God is so good!

This week is a week to praise God. Instead of thinking how scared you may be of labor or fearing how much pain you might have, thank God for giving you this wonderful experience and tell Him you can't wait to meet your baby. He will bless you beyond measure. He has great blessings in store for you. Let's praise Him and give Him all the glory.

Lord, this week, I am feeling and thinking about:

_____

_____

_____

_____

_____

_____

_____

What are You saying to me?

_____

_____

_____

_____

_____

_____

_____

Lord, I am so excited to meet my baby soon. What do You want to tell me before my child arrives?

_____

_____

_____

_____

_____

_____

The first three things I plan to do when I get home with my new baby:

_____

_____

_____

_____

_____

This week, I release to God my cares and concerns about:

_____

_____

_____

_____

_____

_____

_____

_____

_____

_____

_____

_____

_____

## A Mother's Prayer for Week 39

Dear Lord,

I come to You this week with praise in my heart. I know that Your gracious hand is upon me, as Nehemiah 2:18 says. I know You will bless this delivery, Lord. I know that my labor will be manageable, and You will be with me the whole time. Please take away any fear that I may have, and help this baby to come quickly and safely.

You are a great and powerful God. I know that if I praise You, You will rain down Your blessings from above. I believe that You are the Alpha and the Omega, the Beginning and the End. This is a new beginning for my baby, for our family. We praise You for this wonderful gift. Thank You, Heavenly Father.

In Jesus' name. Amen.

# Week 40

Be still before the Lord
and wait patiently for him.
Psalm 37:7 NIV

As you're getting ready to welcome your new baby into your home, I'd like to share with you some tips on having easier labor and delivery. Every woman is unique, so pick and choose the ones you like—and always follow your doctor's advice.

## Ten Tips for Having a Good Labor and Delivery Experience

1. Let go of fear. Stress, tension, and fear make pain worse, so there's no sense in holding on to those negative emotions. Trust is a choice. We can choose to say no to worry and yes to placing our trust in the Lord. This week is a good time to meditate on Scriptures like Proverbs 3:5–6.

2. Concentrate on the positive. "I am getting better at relaxing." "Labor is a natural process." "I can do this; the Lord is by my side." Speaking positive affirmations goes a long way toward having a better birth experience.

3. Have a good coach. Having the support of someone who helps you relax, stay positive, and do the breathing techniques is one of the best secrets for having a good labor experience.

4. Use the breathing techniques. Practice the ones you learned in childbirth class or looked up online. They really do help.

5. Be mobile. Many women find they are better able to deal with contractions by pacing around rather than lying down, as this gives them a greater sense of being in control. Movement also

helps relax the muscles and can prevent you from feeling too tense. I walked the halls in the hospital in my gowns or bounced on a fitness ball to try to get the baby moving, and the contractions weren't nearly as intense as when I was lying down.

6. Try warm water. Some women prefer to sit in a warm tub or to take a shower during labor.

7. Use massage therapy. Have your husband, doula, or coach provide massage therapy with a firm touch. You can use almond oil or your favorite lotion. I know I wouldn't have made it through the 30-plus hours of natural labor if it weren't for my doula massaging my back during each contraction.

8. Try squatting down, sitting up slightly, or another position. For me, squatting in a plié during contractions made me feel better.

9. Listen to Spirit-filled music. God gave us music to lift us up. He dwells in the praises of His people, so worship music brings the Holy Spirit into the room.

10. Have prayer support. Make a list of people who will agree to pray for you while you're in labor and delivery.

Up to now, you've been praying for your unborn baby, and very soon that changes. You will be praying for your son or daughter. Since you've built a good habit of praying for the past nine months, you're in a good position to continue your intercessory prayer ministry for your child. I believe that a mother's job of praying for her children never ends—at least not on this side of Heaven.

Now, let's pray for God's help with your labor and delivery.

Lord, this week, I am feeling and thinking about:

_____

_____

_____

_____

_____

_____

What are You saying to me?

_____

_____

_____

_____

_____

_____

_____

Here is my "mother's blessing" that I pray over my child today:

This week, I release to God my cares and concerns about:

## A Mother's Prayer for Week 40

Dear Lord,

This week is my due date. I thank You for helping me make it to full term in my pregnancy. I am looking forward to welcoming my baby into our home. Lord, please help my baby come at just the right time. Bless my labor and delivery. Give the medical staff wisdom to make all the right decisions. Help me be strong during delivery. Help me trust in You. I pray that Your sweet presence would fill the room with joy as I deliver the baby and we welcome him or her into this world.

Lord, I know You are a good God, and I choose to put my trust in You. Be with me now and every moment of the day. Let me be aware of Your presence with me. Reveal Yourself more to me so I can know You and love You more. Thank You, Lord.

In Jesus' name. Amen.

# Week 41

That you may be filled with the knowledge of His will in all wisdom and spiritual understanding, so that you may walk worthy of the Lord, fully pleasing to Him, bearing fruit in every good work and growing in the knowledge of God. May you be strengthened with all power, according to His glorious might, for all endurance and patience, with joy giving thanks to the Father, who has enabled you to share in the saints' inheritance in the light.

Colossians 1:9–12

Every baby comes on his or her own schedule, and this week, you might still be waiting for your baby to make an appearance. As you wait, here are some Scriptures to reflect and meditate upon:

He will yet fill your mouth with laughter
and your lips with a shout of joy.

Job 8:21

The LORD is my strength and my shield;
my heart trusts in Him, and I am helped.
Therefore my heart rejoices,
and I praise Him with my song.

Psalm 28:7

Lord, this week, I am feeling and thinking about:

What are You saying to me?

This week, I release to God my cares and concerns about:

_____

_____

_____

_____

_____

_____

_____

_____

_____

_____

_____

_____

_____

## A Mother's Prayer for Week 41

Dear Lord,

You know when this baby is ready, and I will praise Your name. I have been waiting for what seems like forever. I feel so uncomfortable and truly can't wait much longer to meet my baby. Please make it happen soon. I know You have a reason for this delay, maybe a miscalculation on the date or maybe my baby's lungs need to mature a bit longer. Whatever it may be, I trust in You, God, and praise Your mighty name.

Jesus, give me peace and rest during these last days before the baby arrives. Make this baby healthy and strong. Please bring the right people to help me deliver this baby. Please let me have this baby in the way I wish, and in the way that's best for him or her, whether natural or C-section. You know what is right for me and my baby. You are a great and wonderful God who has given me a beautiful gift: the gift of life.

I praise Your name, Jesus. Amen.

# Your Hospital Checklist

*What to Take to the Hospital*

This is in printable form at PrayForYourBaby.com.

Time to get ready!

This is a good time to make a list. That way, you won't forget something essential like your camera when that big day finally comes. Consider packing your bag to take to the hospital or birthing center early, just in case your baby decides to surprise you with an early debut!

## For You

- ☐ A comfortable gown
- ☐ Nighttime sanitary napkins
- ☐ A top to wear when visitors come to take pictures
- ☐ Hairbrush or comb, hair clips or hair tie, toothbrush, toothpaste, lip moisturizer, and other personal toiletries
- ☐ Camera and video camera fully charged (and extra batteries just in case)
- ☐ Cell phone and phone numbers

☐ Bible

☐ Spirit-filled music on your playlist

☐ Water and/or Gatorade or Recharge for you and your support team (after you check in at the hospital, they usually won't let you eat)

☐ Stretchy, comfortable clothes to wear home, such as sweatpants, a T-shirt, and socks

☐ Flip-flops or easy slide-in shoes that can get wet

☐ Clothes for your baby to wear home

☐ Baby blankets

☐ Baby car seat for travel home (required)

☐ Copies of your birth plan

☐ Focal point, such as a picture, a prayer, or a small piece of artwork

☐ Mouth spray

☐ Lollipops

☐ Massage tools or a tennis ball

☐ Rice sock heat pack

☐ Ice pack

☐ Lotion, powder, or cornstarch for massage

☐ Fan

☐ Juice ice cubes (or popsicles), juices, sodas

☐ Glasses if you wear contacts

☐ Old pillows that can be washed

☐ Vanilla and/or lavender fragrances

☐ List of who to call

☐ Two small, hard rubber combs (for pressing into palms)

☐ Birth ball

## For Your Partner

- ☐ Snacks and drinks
- ☐ Swimsuit, in case he needs to help you in the shower
- ☐ Change of clothes
- ☐ Toothbrush and toothpaste

## After Birth

- ☐ Nightgown that will make it easy to nurse your baby
- ☐ Robe
- ☐ Nursing bras and pads
- ☐ Breast pump
- ☐ Slippers
- ☐ Makeup